Navigating the Challenges
of Concussion

David C. Spencer, MD, FAAN

Editor, *Brain & Life*® Books Series
Professor of Neurology
Oregon Health and Science University
Portland, OR

Other Titles in the *Brain & Life*® Books Series

Navigating the Challenges of Concussion

Michael S. Jaffee, MD, FAAN, FANA

Professor and Vice-Chair, Department of Neurology
Director, Brain Injury, Rehabilitation, and Neuroresilience (BRAIN) Center
Bob Paul Family Endowed Professor of Neurology
University of Florida

Donna K. Broshek, PhD, ABPP-CN

John Edward Fowler Professor of Psychology
Director, Neuropsychology Assessment Clinic
Co-Director, Acute Concussion Evaluation Clinic, Neurology
University of Virginia Health

Adrian M. Svingos, PhD

Neuropsychologist and Research Scientist
Brain Injury Clinical Research Center
Kennedy Krieger Institute
Baltimore, MD

OXFORD
UNIVERSITY PRESS

OXFORD
UNIVERSITY PRESS

Oxford University Press is a department of the University of Oxford. It furthers
the University's objective of excellence in research, scholarship, and education
by publishing worldwide. Oxford is a registered trade mark of Oxford University
Press in the UK and certain other countries.

Published in the United States of America by Oxford University Press
198 Madison Avenue, New York, NY 10016, United States of America.

Library of Congress Cataloging-in-Publication Data
Names: Jaffee, Michael S., author. | Broshek, Donna K., author. |
Svingos, Adrian M., author.
Title: Navigating the challenges of concussion / Michael S. Jaffee, Donna K. Broshek,
and Adrian M. Svingos.
Other titles: Brain & life* books series.
Description: New York, NY : Oxford University Press, [2023] |
Series: Brain & life books series | Includes bibliographical references and index.
Identifiers: LCCN 2022037295 (print) | LCCN 2022037296 (ebook) |
ISBN 9780190630119 (paperback) | ISBN 9780190630133 (epub) |
ISBN 9780197500033
Subjects: MESH: Brain Concussion—diagnosis |
Brain Concussion—therapy | Popular Work
Classification: LCC RC394.C7 (print) | LCC RC394.C7 (ebook) |
NLM WL 354 | DDC 617.4/81044—dc23/eng/20221109
LC record available at https://lccn.loc.gov/2022037295
LC ebook record available at https://lccn.loc.gov/2022037296

DOI: 10.1093/med/9780190630119.001.0001

This material is not intended to be, and should not be considered, a substitute for medical or
other professional advice. Treatment for the conditions described in this material is highly
dependent on individual circumstances. And, while this material is designed to offer accurate
information with respect to the subject matter covered and to be current as of the time it was
written, research and knowledge about medical and health issues is constantly evolving and
dose schedules for medications are being revised continually, with new side effects recognized
and accounted for regularly. Readers must therefore always check the product information and
clinical procedures with the most up-to-date published product information and data sheets
provided by the manufacturers and the most recent codes of conduct and safety regulation. The
publisher and the authors make no representations or warranties to readers, express or implied,
as to the accuracy or completeness of this material. Without limiting the foregoing, the publisher
and the authors make no representations or warranties as to the accuracy or efficacy of the drug
dosages mentioned in the material. The authors and the publisher do not accept, and expressly
disclaim, any responsibility for any liability, loss or risk that may be claimed or incurred as a
consequence of the use and/or application of any of the contents of this material.

1 3 5 7 9 8 6 4 2
Printed by Sheridan Books, Inc., United States of America

CONTENTS

ABOUT THE *BRAIN & LIFE*®
BOOKS SERIES

What was the first thing you thought when you learned you or a family member had a neurologic condition? Perhaps you were confused, uncertain, afraid, or maybe even in denial. A common thread is often the realization that life has changed and may continue to change, but also uncertainty about exactly what that means or what to expect. And yet, neurologic conditions themselves inevitably change—sometimes quickly, in a matter of seconds or minutes, and sometimes gradually over months or even years.

With any new diagnosis—especially one that is potentially life-changing—you may not be prepared to take in and process large amounts of new information on the spot. And even under the best circumstances, each condition comes with the need to learn a new language and understand the necessary tests, underlying causes, and right treatments. It may be difficult to wrap your arms around a great deal of information in what are often time-limited appointments with your neurologist. Understanding your new diagnosis and how to manage it is a gradual process, and you will inevitably have questions with the passage of time and reflection. Learning about your condition can help you understand what the most useful and accurate information is to share with your neurology team, allowing you to fully participate in treatment decisions.

But facts and information are only part of the picture. You may have questions about how to manage your day-to-day life with a neurologic condition: whether in terms of your career, your home, your relationships, or, in some instances, long-term planning and care. We designed the *Brain & Life* Books series to help you address some of the fears, concerns, and difficult emotions you may feel, such as grief and worry, by harnessing the power of accurate and timely information to help guide you and your family through the change brought about by a neurologic diagnosis. The books share stories of others who have traveled down paths like the one you are on to reinforce the fact that you are not alone.

We selected the authors of the series carefully with these goals in mind. First and foremost, all authors are respected experts in their field, and the information in the *Brain & Life* Books series is accurate, up-to-date, and written to be understandable to someone with no medical background. Experts from the premier neurology organization in the world—the American Academy of Neurology—and the oldest and largest university press in the world—Oxford University Press—carefully review each book to ensure the highest quality. But we also chose our authors because of their experience and ability to connect with patients and their families. The experiences and feelings you are having now have been dealt with and managed successfully by our authors and their patients. Our authors will share with you best practices, stories, and pearls of advice that will leave you with a feeling that your diagnosis is manageable—you can do this. We have highlighted all key terms that you and your family should know when first used, and we have included them in a comprehensive glossary at the back of the book.

The *Brain & Life* Books series was written with you in mind, whether you have been diagnosed yourself or are a family member, caregiver, or friend of someone who has been, as a resource for successfully navigating life with a neurologic condition.

David Spencer, MD, FAAN
Editor, *Brain & Life*® Books
Professor of Neurology
Oregon Health and Science University, Portland, OR

LIST OF FIGURES

PREFACE

Healing is a matter of time, but it is sometimes also a matter of opportunity.

—Hippocrates

Concussion is a mild traumatic brain injury that typically causes temporary symptoms, such as headaches, changes in thinking, dizziness, irritability, and changes in vision. It is a rather common health condition, with between 1.4 million and 3.8 million concussions occurring each year in the United States, according to the U.S. Centers for Disease Control and Prevention. Concussions affect people of all age groups and backgrounds and can occur in many settings and situations. This injury can make it difficult to feel like yourself, think like yourself, or interact with the world as you typically would. Although most people will experience resolution of concussion symptoms within weeks to months, some individuals may experience prolonged symptoms. Even if for a short time, the consequences of the injury can negatively impact work, school, sport, or social activities.

Research suggests that one of the best ways to manage concussion is through education. If you receive appropriate education about the nature of your injury and what to expect with your recovery, you will likely have a better postinjury outcome than someone who does not receive such education. In a world where conversations about concussion have dramatically increased in recent years, receiving accurate, relevant, and individualized information following a concussion is absolutely critical. In addition, knowledge about concussion evaluation and management has been changing rapidly, and not all health care providers may be aware of the latest clinical guidelines. The goal of this book is to help sort through the confusing information in many public sources and older conventional wisdom that you may hear from friends and family so that you can better understand concussion and know what to expect if you or a loved one has one.

Navigating the Challenges of Concussion provides you and your family with facts, patient stories, and helpful guidance about managing the symptoms of concussion and promoting recovery. The book is organized into four main parts. Importantly, the first section will define and clarify what a concussion is and provides information about how concussions can happen, the types of symptoms someone with concussion may experience, and how to facilitate a smooth recovery. It should be reassuring to know that most individuals with a concussion have a good recovery within the expected time frame. It can certainly be quite uncomfortable and stressful to have a concussion. The uncomfortable symptoms feel worse right after the concussion and then gradually improve until you are back to yourself again. Section 1 also provides information on understanding and coping with these typical concussion symptoms.

If your symptoms do not seem to improve or are persisting beyond the typical recovery period, it is important to understand that there may be unique and specific reasons for the persisting symptoms and that these symptoms can be treated. The second section of this book focuses on persisting symptoms after concussion and the various treatments that are available. Some of the recommendations may sound similar to those in earlier chapters, but the focus is on helping you cope with symptoms that do not seem to be getting better as quickly as you had hoped.

The third section discusses special considerations for individuals who may be at increased risk for concussion, including children and adolescents, athletes, military personnel, and older adults, and provides information about returning to school, sports, or work after a concussion.

The fourth and final section discusses the evolution of research in the area of concussion and outlines key questions that researchers and clinicians may attempt to answer in in the future in order to progress scientific understanding and best support individuals affected by concussion.

If you or a loved one have been struggling with a concussion or you are worried about concussion symptoms, it is hoped that this book will increase your understanding of what to expect, clarify misconceptions, and help you feel more hopeful and optimistic about your recovery.

ACKNOWLEDGMENTS

As clinicians who work with people who have experienced concussions, we have seen how overwhelming it can feel to experience a concussion, especially when faced with confusing and contradictory clinical recommendations. Two of us (MJ and DKB) started a multidisciplinary concussion clinic in 2014 to clarify and unify recommendations to patients experiencing an atypical recovery. The following year, we proposed the idea of this patient resource guide to the American Academy of Neurology (AAN) to help demystify concussion and provide practical, evidence-based advice about managing recovery. When Dr. Jaffee moved to Florida in 2016, he started another multidisciplinary clinic and had the good fortune to partner with Dr. Svingos. Together, the authors have treated thousands of patients and have seen how much they benefit from a greater understanding of their symptoms after concussion; these experiences motivated us to write *Navigating the Challenges of Concussion*.

We are indebted to the outstanding editorial team at Oxford University Press headed by Craig Panner for reviewing countless drafts of this book and for providing helpful feedback and guidance each step of the way. We are also grateful to the AAN team of Dr. David Spencer, Andrea Weiss, and Debra Zoellmer for their thoughtful commentary and their detailed feedback, which significantly improved this patient-centered guide.

We are grateful to Dr. George Ansoanuur and Dr. Hunaid Hasan, who took the time to read and provide helpful commentary on earlier drafts of this book while completing busy neurotrauma fellowships. We also appreciate the feedback provided by Matthew Osborne, who read each chapter in detail and provided exceptionally helpful comments on everything from content and phrasing to grammatical style. Merry Kelty read the first few chapters and her perspective also improved the book. We are thankful to Kate Casey-Sawicki, who was instrumental in helping with the arduous task of obtaining proper permissions for the figures.

We are grateful to many mentors and colleagues, but foremost among these is Dr. Jeff Barth. In addition to being a compassionate clinician and educator, Dr. Barth was a vocal advocate for patients who sustained brain injuries. He brought attention to the challenges experienced by patients who had mild brain injuries well before many other professionals recognized these problems. Widely recognized as the father of sports neuropsychology, Dr. Barth and his colleagues at the University of Virginia were the first to demonstrate that cognitive symptoms occurred in football players after a concussion, that these symptoms could be measured, and that the players recovered. On a personal note, Dr. Barth is a truly kind and caring person with nonstop good humor. He is both a mentor and beloved friend and colleague.

We would also like to offer our gratitude to Dr. Rus Bauer, who has been a true advocate and leader in the field and has offered his wisdom, leadership, and advice to the Department of Defense. He has made many contributions to the field of neuropsychology, including as Past-President of the International Neuropsychological Society and as a member of the Board of the American Academy of Clinical Neuropsychology. He is an unparalleled clinical neuropsychologist and researcher of the highest caliber who has educated generations of neurologists and neuropsychologists. Dr. Bauer has been a visionary partner, colleague, and role model.

Each of us experienced many life changes and challenges while writing this book, and we are grateful for the support of our families.

Through the love and encouragement of his family, Dr. Jaffee was able to navigate unexpected health challenges while balancing professional duties. His wife, Michelle, both a professional writer and his personal muse, has exemplified boundless dedication and tenderness—she is truly his "media naranja." His twin daughters, Clara and Tessa, have matured into naturally compassionate and empathetic young women; they are both a source of deep pride and inspiration. While writing this book, Dr. Jaffee also lost his father, Dr. I. Sidney Jaffee, "the OG Dr. Jaffee"—the quintessential beneficent physician. He relished not only helping others as an ENT doctor but also truly connecting with his patients. He taught Dr. M. Jaffee the value of learning everyone's story.

After a period of extended caregiving, Dr. Broshek lost her mother, Lora Rebecca "Becky" Broshek, during the first year of writing this book. Her mother was pure sunshine and taught the importance of appreciating others as well as small moments of beauty. After this difficult loss, Dr. Broshek received the gift of meeting her best friend, Dr. Bill Fox, and they eloped during the pandemic. She would like to express her gratitude to her husband for his love, support, kindness, and unfailing good humor. And Dr. Broshek is also grateful to her sisters, Pat Verdugo, Jacky Copeland, and Sandy Enyeart, for all the years of love, support, and laughter and for her wonderful nieces and nephews.

Dr. Svingos' contributions to the work would not have been possible without the support of family and most of all her husband, Robert "Sotiri," whose spirit of patience and love are unparalleled. She would like to thank her precious daughters, Elizabeth "Vetta" and Vaia, for their amazing napping tendencies during infancy and for the unmeasurable joy and inspiration that they provided as this book took form during their earliest months and years.

We learn as we treat. We are grateful for our fellows, residents, students, and trainees who have helped shape our learning communities. We gain knowledge from each patient and are dedicated to growing as health professionals who can best serve those affected by concussion. We would like to thank each of our patients and research participants for sharing their stories—and for inspiring the work that we do each day. Thank you for allowing us to be a part of your journey.

Concussion and Typical Recovery

What Is a Concussion?

In this chapter, you will learn:

- What a concussion is and how it occurs
- How a concussion is different from other types of head injuries
- The initial signs and symptoms of concussion

In general, **concussion** is a temporary change in brain functioning, or the ability of the brain to do its job, when forces from an impact (e.g., a fall) or other type of injury reach the brain. We will explain more about the medical definition of concussion later in this chapter. Concussions can occur in any number of ways; the most common are falls; motor vehicle accidents; sports-related injuries; and recreational activities such as biking, skateboarding, or skiing. Concussions can result from direct impact (i.e., hitting your head hard against an object) or indirect impact (taking a hit to another part of your body with a force strong enough to reach your brain).

So What Really Happens?

So how does concussion affect your brain? Your brain can be thought of as the control center for the rest of your body, with different parts of the brain working together to help you think and understand information, carry out controlled movement (such as walking), experience emotions, or speak. The brain communicates and coordinates these functions through a precise balance of chemicals. To carry out all these different functions, your brain also needs energy (which is supplied by **glucose**). When you experience a hard hit or jarring impact, **biomechanical forces** are transmitted to the brain, disrupting the natural balance of chemicals. This is a concussion.

Your brain will work hard to try to restore its normal functioning and communicate that more energy is needed to maintain that function. Normal blood flow in the brain is also altered, which makes it harder for the cells to deliver this needed energy. So early in this process when the brain needs more energy, it experiences a period of reduced energy. The increased energy demand and reduced energy supply create a mismatch that generally lasts 1 to 4 weeks in adults and usually closer to 4 weeks for children and adolescents. This period of energy depletion in the brain is common in all types of concussions and is typically associated with symptoms such as headaches, concentration difficulties, vision disturbance, dizziness, and difficulty in controlling emotions. As the brain begins to return to normal function, concussion symptoms start to resolve. Let's use some case examples to explore how different causes of concussion can further affect the brain.

Causes of Concussion

Jasmine is in her car when she rear-ends another car at a red light. Upon impact, her head quickly whips forward and then back again. Her airbag does not go off, and her head does not hit any part of the car or any objects within the car because she is wearing her seat belt. She is, however, startled by what happened, and when she looks up, her vision is blurry and she feels rather nauseous. She is taken to the hospital for evaluation, and medical evaluation determines that she has a concussion.

The brain sits in fluid inside the skull, and when the head moves rapidly back and forth on the neck, the brain moves around inside the skull and a concussion can occur. This type of injury, called an **acceleration–deceleration injury**, is what happened to Jasmine in the patient story. As you recall, she did not hit her head or body on any part of the car, but the force of the collision pushed her head rapidly forward and then backward. You may also hear this type of injury referred to as a **whiplash injury**.

> *John is knocked out with a swift right hook to the jaw during his last boxing match. A few minutes later, he wakes up and is noticeably irritable, insisting that the match has not yet started. Upon reviewing film with his coach, John sees that his opponent had delivered a quick horizontal punch to his jaw, causing his head to rapidly shift backward before he fell to the ground.*

Some concussions occur as a result of rotational forces, sometimes referred to as **rotational injury**. Rotational injuries occur when forces hitting the head or body cause the head and neck to forcefully turn to one side. When the head rotates on the neck, the brain moves in an arc inside the skull and bundles of **brain fibers** (also known as **axons**) that connect one part of the brain with another part for communication can be stretched or sheared, which can result in a loss of consciousness or change in mental status (like John's irritability) or functioning. Axons are the parts of a brain cell that transmit information. They often bundle together to create **tracts** ("information highways") for communication among different parts of the brain.

Injuries caused by very strong forces, such as those in high-speed car accidents or a knockout punch, sometimes can result in the stretching or shearing of axons within the brain. This type of injury, referred to as **diffuse axonal injury**, usually only occurs when very strong forces are transmitted to the brain, including both forces that make the head and neck increase in speed and then rapidly decrease in speed (acceleration–deceleration injury) and those that make the head turn quickly (rotational forces).

Concussion can also occur as a result of forces that are produced after an explosion. These types of injuries, called **blast injuries**, are common in military personnel who are exposed to explosions during combat or training. Blast injuries and some of the unique challenges experienced by military personnel with concussion are discussed in Chapter 14.

How Is Concussion Different from Other Forms of Head Injury?

Before we get into the specifics of the symptoms you might experience with concussion, let's first clarify some terms used to describe injuries involving the brain or head. **Head injury** is a general term used to describe any injury to the scalp, head, or brain. **Brain injury** is also a general term and is used to describe an insult or injury from any cause specifically involving the brain. A **traumatic brain injury** is a specific form of brain injury caused by physical trauma.

Traumatic brain injuries are typically divided into **mild, moderate,** or **severe traumatic brain injury.** Over the years, medical providers and researchers have developed ways of distinguishing mild from moderate and severe traumatic brain injuries based on symptoms that tend to be associated with prognosis or outcome. People with mild traumatic brain injuries tend to have a much better recovery than those with more severe injuries. If you have had a concussion, you may have heard your doctor refer to your injury as a **mild traumatic brain injury** because these terms generally mean the same thing. Concussions are considered mild forms of traumatic brain injury because they change the way the brain works for a temporary period of time and the symptoms of concussion (or mild traumatic brain injury) are expected to improve over time. Although some factors can prolong or complicate concussion recovery (see Chapters 7 and 8), concussion typically does not cause permanent brain damage nor does it result in significant disability as more severe brain injuries can.

Although this book focuses solely on concussion, it is important to briefly explain the more severe forms of traumatic brain injury so you understand the differences, which will be helpful when you discuss your injury with your primary care physician and other health care providers. Signs that suggest you may have had a moderate or severe traumatic brain injury (which are more severe than a concussion) include:

- Losing consciousness for longer than 30 minutes
- Having difficulty forming new memories (called **posttraumatic amnesia**) for more than a day
- Significant difficulties on a measure called the **Glasgow Coma Scale (GCS)**

While not a diagnostic tool, the GCS is a score used by **emergency medical technicians** (EMTs) and medical staff in an emergency department to estimate the severity of a brain injury. The GCS score ranges from 3 to 15 and is based on symptoms related to eye opening, verbal responses, and **motor functioning**. A low score suggests that a person is not responding at all or that their functioning is very impaired, while a high score reflects more minimal injury. If injured, scores in the 13 to 15 range on the GCS typically reflect a mild traumatic brain injury or concussion. Scores lower than 13 typically indicate a moderate or more severe traumatic brain injury that needs medical attention right away. You may see this score in your medical records or hear your health care providers talk about this score as an indicator that you did not have a more severe injury.

Niko and Tara are driving home from visiting with friends when they are involved in a high-speed collision on the highway. Niko is driving and is not restrained, whereas Tara is in the passenger seat and is wearing her seat belt. In the collision, Niko is ejected from the vehicle, flying through the windshield and landing almost 15 feet away from the car. Tara loses consciousness for several minutes. When she comes to, EMTs have safely extracted her from the vehicle; they conduct an assessment of her level of awareness and note that she is somewhat confused and not fully oriented. The EMTs assign her a GCS score of 14 out of 15, suggesting that she has sustained a mild traumatic brain injury or concussion. She has several lacerations and is taken to the hospital for ongoing evaluation and monitoring. Niko is in extremely critical condition, and she is told that he has survived but is completely unresponsive (with a GCS score of 3 out of 15), representing the most severe form of traumatic brain injury. Niko is having trouble breathing on his own, and the EMTs on the scene have to place a breathing tube through his mouth and into his windpipe (intubation) so they can support his breathing and transport him to the hospital, where he is admitted to the intensive care unit. Tara recovers from her concussion over the course of the following week, whereas Niko remains in a vegetative state for 2 months and requires supportive care for the remainder of his life because of significant cognitive and physical disability.

People are sometimes confused by the terminology and classification of traumatic brain injury as mild, moderate, and severe. It is important to remember that this classification does not refer to the severity of your current symptoms but rather the characteristics of your initial injury. Having a concussion means that your prognosis is better than someone with a more severe form of traumatic brain injury, but it does not mean that your symptoms will necessarily feel "mild."

Another area of confusion is that mild traumatic brain injury can be a very broad classification that includes those who do not have a loss of consciousness and who are able to talk and move freely after their injury, as well as those who have a 20–29 minute loss of consciousness and are confused and disoriented for up to 24 hours. Some people diagnosed with a mild traumatic brain injury might even have small brain bleeds. As you can see this is a very broad range of severity within the category of "mild" traumatic brain injury. When research groups everyone with a mild brain injury together, the research findings may be confusing and suggest that everyone with a mild traumatic brain injury may have persisting symptoms over a long period of time. Different scientific and medical organizations use different definitions to categorize these injuries so it is important to talk to your health care provider to understand the specifics of your brain injury.

Now you know how concussion is different from more severe forms of brain injury, but how is it different from other, more minor, forms of head injury? Some people may experience hits to their head in their daily life, such as bumping their head on a cabinet door or doorframe, but neither of these minor hits cause concussions. The human skull is quite strong and durable and protects our brains from many types of minor impacts such as hitting a doorframe. A hit to the head can cause a brief jolt of pain and may result in an area of tenderness or even swelling, but if you have no acute symptoms such as feeling confused or dazed, it is probably not a concussion. You might even hit your head hard enough to have bleeding from your scalp or significant swelling on your head (a "goose egg") without having any symptoms indicative of concussion. So, what exactly are the symptoms of concussion?

Acute Signs and Symptoms of Concussion

Tina is a 35-year-old woman who works as a physical therapist at the local hospital and enjoys her job. She is in excellent cardiovascular health and regularly competes in local half-marathons and marathons. During the final stretch of one of her morning runs, she slips on wet pavement and falls to the ground. She is unable to brace her fall, and her forehead goes straight into the concrete. Tina does not lose consciousness and immediately gets up. She isn't bleeding and decides to continue running. During the next mile, Tina noticed that she feels "a bit off," experiencing mild dizziness and nausea. When she finishes her run, she feels more tired than usual, but she attributes it to having stayed up late the night before. The following day, she has a hard time sticking to her morning routine because simple decisions (e.g., what to pack for lunch) have become more difficult and require more time for her to think through. Tina is late to work that day and has a hard time falling asleep that night. She is still feeling off the next day and describes what had happened to her husband, who is concerned that she may have injured herself in some way. He encourages her to go to the emergency department. Upon evaluation, it is determined that she likely has a concussion. She is given recommendations to promote optimal recovery, is provided with information about what to expect during the recovery process, and is sent home and encouraged to follow up with her primary care physician, if needed.

Some people are unaware that they have had a concussive injury. One person might feel "a bit off," whereas others might feel as if they "had their bell rung" or may recognize more noticeable acute symptoms, such as dizziness, headache, sensitivity to light or sound, or balance problems. It is important to realize that no two brains are exactly alike and that each injury has its own unique mechanism or set of forces that affects brain function. Concussions usually involve a brief change in your ability to think clearly (alteration of consciousness) or, in some cases, a clear loss of consciousness for a short period of time. It is important to note, however, that you can have a concussion without losing consciousness; in fact, most concussions occur without a loss of consciousness.

Although a number of symptoms tend to occur in the context of a concussion, these symptoms typically vary from person to person and may also differ in severity. The most frequently reported symptoms among people who have sustained a concussion include the following:

- Physical symptoms
  - Headache/pressure in head
  - Sensitivity to light
  - Sensitivity to noise
  - Neck pain
  - Nausea/vomiting
  - Blurred vision
  - Balance problems
  - Dizziness
  - Difficulty falling/staying asleep
- Cognitive symptoms
  - Feeling slowed down
  - Feeling in a fog
  - Not feeling right
  - Difficulty concentrating
  - Difficulty remembering
  - Confusion
- Emotional symptoms
  - Feeling irritable
  - Feeling more emotional

- o Feeling sad
- o Feeling nervous/anxious
- o Lack of motivation

You may attribute some of your concussion symptoms to other causes, such as assuming that you feel more tired than usual because you stayed up late. It is not unusual to be unsure whether your symptoms are due to a concussion, as many of the symptoms are not specific to concussion but occur in a variety of health conditions and circumstances, especially when you are under stress or sleep-deprived. You may think it is unlikely that you had a concussion because you did not lose consciousness when you hit your head, but remember, most people who sustain concussions do not experience a loss of consciousness.

Summary

This chapter described how concussion is defined and how it is different from other forms of head injury. It is important to remember that a concussion can occur without a direct hit to the head and that you don't need to lose consciousness to have had a concussion. Concussions usually involve some temporary disruption of thinking skills or brief alteration of awareness, among other symptoms. Concussion has many different acute symptoms, and these same symptoms occur in a variety of health conditions and situations, which can sometimes make concussions difficult to detect. Chapter 2 discusses how medical providers acutely identify and manage concussions.

Assessing and Managing Your Concussion

The Initial Evaluation

In this chapter, you will learn:

- How medical providers acutely manage concussion
- Some of the information that medical providers may share with you immediately following your concussion

Concussion is described by many as an "invisible injury." It is different from a scrape, bruise, or broken limb, where the consequences of injury are visible in plain sight. Concussion causes changes within the brain, as was described in the first chapter, and these changes may not be obvious to others, which can make it difficult for parents, friends, or even some health care providers to really understand what you or your family member may be going through. Despite this, an increasing number of individuals are becoming aware of concussion and its signs and symptoms due to media coverage, advocacy, and state and federal legislation. Similarly, researchers and clinicians who treat patients with concussions have come a long way in their ability to acutely identify and manage concussion to promote optimal recovery. This chapter covers how your doctors or other health care providers may manage your concussion acutely—right after the concussion occurs—to ensure that you are on the right track for a smooth recovery.

What to Expect When You Are Being Evaluated for a Concussion

> *Brandon is a 19-year-old university student pursuing a degree in advertising. He was on his way home from school one afternoon driving at approximately 45 miles per hour when he looked down at his phone to check a text message from a friend. When he looked back up at the road, he saw that the cars in front of him were stopped, and he slammed on his brakes but was not able to brake in time to avoid a collision. Brandon's airbag deployed and his car was totaled. Following the accident, Brandon was confused as to where he was and had a terrible headache. He managed to get out of his car with help from first responders and was taken to the hospital by an ambulance to be evaluated. At the hospital, it was determined that Brandon had sustained a concussion due to rapid acceleration and deceleration, as well as a variety of orthopedic injuries. Brain imaging was negative for any abnormalities, and Brandon was sent home with a prescription for physical therapy and a pamphlet about concussion.*

One of the primary goals of the initial concussion assessment is to ensure that the injured person is safe. Following a head injury, it is important to be evaluated by a medical professional in order to rule out a more serious condition. While an initial evaluation may occur on the scene of an injury by emergency medical technicians (EMTs), in many cases, this initial evaluation takes place in a hospital emergency room or emergency department (ED). If an EMT has already conducted an evaluation of clinical status, this important information, including the Glasgow Coma Scale score, will be provided to the ED physician.

In the ED, a nurse or other member of the medical care team may ask you some questions about your head injury—what happened, when it happened, and what you experienced—and gather details about your medical history and the current symptoms that you are experiencing. An emergency medicine physician may carry out a thorough **neurologic examination** to assess how well your brain is functioning. In some cases, the ED physician may consult with a **neurologist** who is available in the hospital or by phone. This neurologic examination will likely involve checking to see if you are fully **oriented** (e.g., knowing who you are, where you are, and the date/time), that your **cranial nerves** (bundles of brain cells that usually connect with our brainstem and work together to carry out specific functions for our head, face, and special senses) are intact, that your reflexes are working, and that you can coordinate movement and feel sensations appropriately. You may be asked to do some simple calculations in your head, remember some words, or draw a copy of a figure. You may also be asked to walk down a hallway so that the ED physician can see how you are walking. This examination could help your physician rule out a more serious brain injury or provide information that signals a more serious condition.

Depending on the severity of your symptoms, your physician may want to request additional tests in order to provide the right diagnosis and treatment. Although patients with concussions typically do not have their brain scanned in the ED with a head **CT** (**computed tomography scan** of the head), some patients will be asked to undergo a CT scan depending on their symptoms. Symptoms that are not typical of a concussion and may indicate a more severe type of brain injury are called "**red flags.**" Red flags include:

- Decreasing level of alertness
- Increasing confusion
- Severe or rapidly worsening headache
- Repeated vomiting

- Seizures
- Weakness or numbness in the arms or legs
- Eye pupils of unequal size
- Slurred speech or inability to talk
- Inability to recognize people or places
- Persisting double vision
- Loss of part of vision (visual field cut)
- Severe neck pain

In these situations, the ED physician may request that you undergo prompt brain imaging to ensure that there are no active bleeds or evolving changes in your brain that would require an urgent intervention such as neurosurgery. The ED physician may choose to do a CT to quickly rule out a more severe injury. Head CTs can be performed quickly (in around 10 minutes or less) and are capable of detecting major abnormalities within the brain. A CT scanner is shown in Figure 2.1. If the head CT shows changes in the brain that may indicate damage to brain tissue (often called positive **neuroimaging** findings), those findings would typically indicate a brain injury that is more severe than a concussion.

Unfortunately, these scans do expose you to small amounts of radiation because they use **x-ray** technology. The risk of radiation exposure is the reason why not everyone with a concussion automatically has a head CT. Health care providers weigh the costs and benefits of every test; if there is no reason to suspect any brain bleeds or changes in your brain structure, then the risk of radiation exposure outweighs the potential benefit of a scan. If the ED doctor does not identify red flags or have concerns about a more serious injury, it is safer for you not to have a head CT. If you are pregnant or think there is a chance that you might be pregnant, it is important to inform the technician. If the CT scan is completely necessary, extra precautions can be taken to protect the unborn baby from potential exposure to radiation.

It is important to note that medical professionals and researchers are still learning about the best ways to diagnose and manage

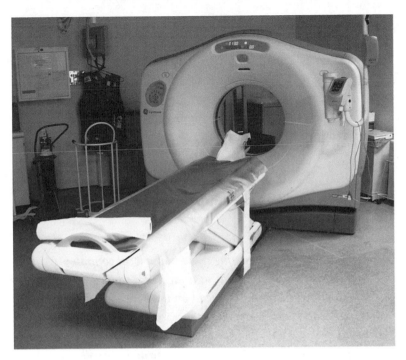

FIGURE 2.1. A typical CT scanner

Originally published in James Thomas and Tanya Monaghan. Oxford Handbook of Clinical Examination and Practical Skills, 2nd ed. Copyright © 2014, Oxford Publishing Limited. DOI: 10.1093/med/9780199593972.001.0001. Reproduced with permission of Oxford Publishing Limited through PLSclear.

concussion effectively during the initial evaluation, or right after a suspected concussion has occurred. One focus of research has been on identifying blood-based **biomarkers** that may help speed up the acute assessment process and determine whether someone has had a concussion. At this time, researchers have found at least two **proteins** in the blood that tend to be elevated when a person has sustained an injury significant enough to be seen on CT scan. These protein markers, called **UCHL-1 and GFAP**, were recently approved by the U.S. Food and Drug Administration (FDA) for clinical use in the ED as markers to help rule out more serious forms of brain injury when assessing for concussion. What this means for the future of concussion assessment is that blood tests may ultimately replace routine brain imaging as a method for ruling out more serious underlying injuries. This could be helpful because blood tests are less expensive than CT scans and do not expose you to any radiation. This is a rapidly growing area of study and more protein markers of brain injury may be identified in the near future.

Getting the Right Information

Cathy is a 23-year-old nursing student at a local community college. She was out with friends at a nightclub when someone accidentally elbowed her in the head on the dance floor. Cathy felt a bit off balance afterwards but otherwise felt okay. She had been drinking and was enjoying herself. The next day, she woke up with a terrible headache and felt nauseous. She had a small bump on her head where she had been elbowed. Cathy's roommate, also a nursing student, saw what had happened the night before and insisted that Cathy had sustained a concussion. She told Cathy that she should stay in a dark room as much as possible in order to help her brain heal faster. She also cautioned Cathy against going to her yoga class, insisting that she eliminate all physical activities for at least 1 month. Cathy did some research online and decided that she should also take a few weeks off from school in order to let her brain heal. When Cathy tried to go back to school, the overhead projector hurt her eyes and she developed a slight headache. Cathy was worried about missing any more class but feared that it could be dangerous for her to stay. About 6 weeks later, Cathy had still not gotten back to school and was starting to feel down. She set up an appointment to be evaluated in a specialty concussion clinic, hoping for some answers.

The amount of accurate information and education you receive right after a suspected concussion can have a substantial impact on your recovery. In our example, Cathy receives inaccurate information from a variety of sources like that from her roommate and online. She was under the impression that she should stay in a dark room and that she should discontinue all physical activities for at least 1 month. This advice is sometimes referred to as "**cocooning**" by health care professionals. The advice is well intended, hoping to protect or "cocoon" the individual from any stimulation that may make symptoms worse. However, our scientific understanding shows that sustained "cocooning" can actually prolong recovery. While every effort should be made to reduce the risk of having a second injury right after a concussion, there is no evidence to suggest that light physical exercise during the first few days after concussion can damage your brain. In fact, evidence has shown just the opposite—that mild (non-contact) exercise right after a concussion can actually promote optimal recovery. Immediately following a concussion, excessive strenuous mental activity, such as extended reading and writing, can worsen symptoms and is most likely not a good thing. Doing "too much" is probably just as bad as doing "too little." In general, it is recommended that you gradually get back to your ordinary life activities, including school or work, as soon as possible, using symptoms as a gauge for the pace at which this should happen. We will discuss specific protocols and recommendations for concussions that occur in sports and military activity as well as returning to school and to work in Section 3 at the end of the book.

Your Concussion Health Care Team

Once you or your child has been definitely diagnosed with a concussion, you can get some guidance on what to do next. Your doctor or health care team can then help you develop a plan for managing any symptoms you may have and for re-entry into your typical activities. You may receive this information in the ED or in an outpatient setting such as with your primary care physician or your child's **pediatrician,** or in an **interdisciplinary concussion clinic.** In an interdisciplinary clinic, you will see a group of medical professionals from different fields—called an **interdisciplinary team**—who work together to provide you with a specialized treatment plan for optimal recovery. Your interdisciplinary team may include providers such as a neurologist, a **physical medicine and rehabilitation (PM&R)** physician (also called a **physiatrist), neuropsychologist, physical therapist,** and **occupational therapist.** These health care professionals will work with you to determine the most appropriate pace for re-entry into life activities based upon your history and symptoms and the findings from their evaluation. Let's talk a little bit more about these specialists, their training, what they do, and their role in your recovery:

- Nursing staff may play a role in obtaining your vital signs (height, weight, blood pressure, temperature) and reviewing your medications, vitamins, or any other supplements you may be taking.
- The neurologist, **advanced practice nurse,** or **physician assistant** will gather information during an interview; will review your medical history, medications, and supplements; and will conduct a thorough physical and neurologic examination.
- The neuropsychologist will gather information during an interview specific to cognitive and emotional functioning and history and may give you questionnaires that ask about aspects of your history and current functioning. They may also administer cognitive tests to provide information about your current thinking skills to track your recovery, provide education, and make recommendations to help you with any thinking difficulties.
- The PM&R physician, often called a physiatrist, is another type of doctor who gathers information about your concussion; reviews your medical history, medications, and supplements;

and conducts a physical examination. They are typically involved when the concussion occurs in a setting of multiple injuries such as from a motor vehicle collision and are skilled in pain management.

- The physical therapist will gather relevant information during a brief interview and will likely put you through physical exertion testing as well as testing of your balance and vision.
- An **occu**pational therapist will assess your functional abilities in areas as basic as self-care to as complex as driving. An occupational therapy assessment will involve an interview portion and may also require you to fill out questionnaires or carry out certain activities to assess your level of abilities. Occupational therapists are experts in understanding how physical, cognitive, or emotional disturbances associated with your injury may be impacting your daily functioning. Some occupational therapists specialize in assessments of eye movements and visual symptoms.

Each of these specialists has specialized training and experience in different aspects of health care, and depending on your particular symptoms, each of them may play an important role in your recovery. Most who experience a concussion recover without seeing these different professionals. If you have a more challenging recovery process, however, you may see some or all of them and they will develop a specific plan based on your specific symptoms to help you feel better.

Summary

In this chapter, we provided information about how medical professionals may evaluate you for concussion, right after an injury. While there is no "one size fits all" method for how concussions are acutely managed, the most important components involve being evaluated quickly and making sure that you get access to accurate and up-to-date information about the initial recovery process. The next three chapters of this book provide a more detailed look at some of the specific symptoms of concussion and how these symptoms may be best managed in order to promote optimal recovery.

Early Physical Symptoms of Concussion

In this chapter, you will learn:

- How concussion can cause physical symptoms
- How your doctor will evaluate you for these symptoms and make recommendations for your treatment

After a concussion, you may experience a broad spectrum of symptoms, both before and after you see your doctor or the emergency department staff. These symptoms may affect your thinking skills or mood or may cause pain or discomfort. Not everyone will have the same symptoms following a concussion, and not everyone will recover at the same rate. This chapter focuses on the physical symptoms of concussion, including headache, dizziness, and sleep problems. The emotional and cognitive symptoms of concussion are discussed in later chapters.

Headaches

Headaches are among the most common symptoms to occur following a concussion. If you start to experience headaches within a week of a concussion, you may have what is sometimes called **post-concussive headaches** or **acute posttraumatic headaches**. Headaches can be debilitating and can make it difficult to concentrate or get enough rest. If you are experiencing post-concussive headaches, it will be important to discuss them with your medical team.

One of the first things your clinician will do is determine the features of the headaches you are experiencing to develop an appropriate treatment strategy. Your doctor will ask you to describe the type of pain you are having and where in your head the pain occurs. For example, is the pain throbbing, stabbing, or burning? Is the pain only on one side of your head? Where specifically are you experiencing the pain? Your doctor will also likely ask about other symptoms that can be associated with headache pain, such as nausea, sensitivity to light, and sensitivity to sounds.

Your clinician will also do a thorough examination to ensure that you have no signs of a more concerning cause of the headaches, such as a brain bleed. This evaluation typically involves a head-to-toe assessment of your functioning. The clinician will look into your eyes with a light and watch you move your eyes to look at a pointer or finger. Just as they did in the emergency department, the clinician evaluating your headaches will observe how you walk, check your strength and coordination, and test your reflexes. If your clinician notices signs that could indicate a possible brain bleed or more severe form of brain injury, they may want you to have neuroimaging with computed tomography (CT) or **magnetic resonance imaging (MRI)**, if neuroimaging was not already performed. A picture of an MRI scanner is shown in Figure 3.1.

Although currently no standardized guidelines have been established for the early management of posttraumatic headache pain, your doctor will make individualized recommendations for you based on your specific injury and current symptoms. For example, if your doctor has ruled out a more significant brain injury (e.g., a brain bleed), they may recommend that you try taking an over-the-counter pain reliever, such as ibuprofen (Advil), acetaminophen (Tylenol), or naproxen (Aleve), to manage headache pain. It is very important that you only take these medications after consulting with your health care provider because some are also blood thinners or medications that could worsen other medical problems, such as kidney disease. It is also important that you only take over-the-counter headache medications under the care of your clinician because taking too many over-the-counter medications can actually

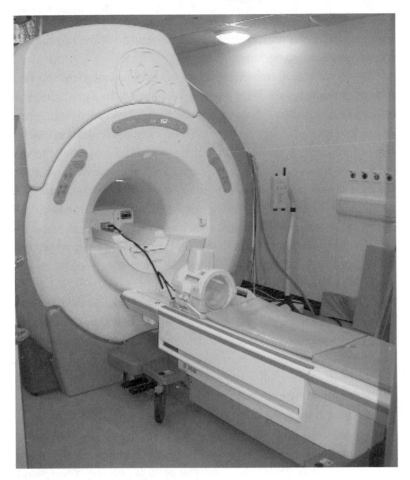

FIGURE 3.1. A typical MRI scanner
Originally published in James Thomas and Tanya Monaghan. Oxford Handbook of
Clinical Examination and Practical Skills, 2nd ed. Copyright © 2014, Oxford Publishing
Limited. DOI: 10.1093/med/9780199593972.001.0001. Reproduced with permission of
Oxford Publishing Limited through PLSclear.

make headaches worse, a phenomenon referred to as **medication-
overuse headaches** or **rebound headaches**. Medication-overuse
headaches tend to feel just like posttraumatic headaches and
thus can be difficult to identify without the help of a physician.

Medications that include caffeine in the ingredients, such as most forms of Excedrin and Fiorinal/Fioricet, tend to have the highest risk for medication-overuse headaches.

As you may recall from Chapter 1, concussions can sometimes result when rapid acceleration and deceleration of the head and neck occur, which is often the case in motor vehicle accidents. In these cases, headache pain can be the result of whiplash injury because of strained muscles in the back of the neck and head. This type of injury has several names, including **cervicalgia** and **cervicogenic headache**. A major sign of cervicalgia is simultaneous headache and neck pain that starts at the time of the injury. Headaches resulting from whiplash can include migraine-like features, such as throbbing pain with nausea and sensitivity to light. These headaches may also be described as a tight band-like sensation around the head, known as **muscle tension headaches** or **tension-type headaches**.

If you are experiencing headache pain after a suspected concussion, your clinician will want to rule out **musculoskeletal** factors that could be contributing to your pain. These factors could include muscle strain, neck injury, or nerve irritation. Your clinician may prescribe topical medications such as a cream or gel to help the tightened muscles relax, providing pain relief to the affected area. They may also prescribe **physical therapy** or alternative treatments, such as massage, to relieve pain. Providers who do not explicitly specialize in concussion may sometimes miss a neck injury, which can complicate the recovery process because of prolonged headache pain. If you are experiencing headache and neck pain after a suspected concussion, it is important to ask your medical provider to rule out an underlying neck injury and communicate all relevant information regarding your injury, including specific information about the type of pain you are experiencing. Chapter 7 provides more information about specific treatment options for headache pain, including **cervicogenic headache**, in the more chronic phase (months after a concussion has occurred).

If you struggled with migraines or other headache syndromes before your concussion occurred, a few other important things should be taken into consideration. A concussion can trigger or worsen these headaches, even if they were previously under control with medications. It is important to discuss with your clinician any medications for headache or migraine you were taking before your concussion. In most cases, your physician will recommend that you continue with your preexisting medication regimen. However, it is critical that you undergo an evaluation by a health care provider so that they can pinpoint the cause of the worsening preexisting headache.

If your headaches are found to be consistent with **migraine,** your doctor may recommend that you use **rescue medication** for migraine. These medications may include **triptans** such as **suma-triptan** (Imitrex), rizatriptan (Maxalt), and zolmitriptan (Zomig). These medications target the chemical messenger neurotransmitter **serotonin** by attaching to the specialized receptors that exist for this chemical on blood vessels and **nerve cells** and reduce the enlargement of brain blood vessels that can occur during a migraine. The effect of this medication on nerve cells is to slow down or stop the release of **inflammatory proteins,** such as **Substance P** and **calcitonin gene-related peptide (CGRP),** which would sustain a migraine. Each of these inflammatory proteins binds to its own nerve cell receptors to cause a cascade of release of the inflammatory agents. The reduced release of Substance P and CGRP helps stop this **inflammatory cascade** and thus helps to stop a headache. One concern with the triptan medications is that they can constrict blood vessels, so this may not be a safe option for those with heart or vascular disease.

New headache medications that may be helpful for patients struggling with migraines that are made worse by a concussion continue to be developed. A new class of medications called **calcitonin gene-related peptide receptor antagonists,** or **CGRP inhibitors,** have recently been made available. These medications target the inflammatory process described above. There are two types of medicines within this new class that work in different ways to prevent an inflammatory cascade. One type uses antibodies that target CGRP proteins before they bind to the nerve cell and then activate an inflammatory cascade. Because these medications have a long effect over time (long half-life), they are typically administered by injection once per month and are used as part of a regimen for more chronic or persistent headache syndromes. These longer-acting medications include erenumab (Aimovig), galcanezumab (Emgality), fremanezumab (Ajovy), and eptinezumab (Vyepti).

The other type of medication within this class binds the CGRP receptor directly on the nerve cell, blocking its use by a CGRP protein and thus preventing the inflammatory cascade. Because they have smaller molecules, these medications are typically taken as pills and work faster for a shorter period of time. These medications may be used for rapid relief of headache pain. These include ubrogepant (Ubrelvy) and rimegepant (Nurtec). Unlike triptans, these new medications do not constrict blood vessels and thus can be used in patients with heart or vascular disease.

If you are experiencing significant migraine pain that impairs your day-to-day functioning, your doctor may also add other medications to break the migraine cycle. These may include a scheduled brief course of medications that can reduce inflammation within the body such as **steroids** (prednisone) or **nonsteroidal anti-inflammatory drugs** (**NSAIDs**) at prescription doses, such as naproxen. Alternatively, your physician may prescribe an **atypical neuroleptic medication** such as olanzapine (Zyprexa) to break the cycle using a regimen found to be effective in treating sustained migraine syndromes. It is thought that the use of these medications for a brief period of time can help break the migraine cycle by reducing inflammation within the brain or targeting the migraine generator in the brainstem.

If you continue to experience headaches after your other concussion symptoms have resolved, you may benefit from the additional recommendations described in Chapter 7.

Dizziness and Balance Problems

> *Brian is a college student who is out with friends on Saturday night when he finds himself in the middle of an argument that becomes physical. He ends up taking a punch that knocks him out for a few seconds. He goes to the emergency department, where he is diagnosed with a concussion and encouraged to follow up at the student health care center on Monday. He is sitting in the dining hall the following morning when he notices the room seems to be spinning around him. He feels very sick to his stomach and as though he needs to hold on to the table or he'll fall over. His friend helps him back to his dorm room, where he is able to rest until the spinning sensation becomes less intense. When he is evaluated the following day, he undergoes a maneuver called the **Dix-Hallpike** that requires him to lie face up on an exam table with his head hanging over the edge of the table. This immediately brings back the intense spinning sensation, and he feels very ill. His doctor then performs a maneuver in which he holds Brian's head in various positions for timed intervals. The doctor shows him how to carry out this procedure at home to improve his symptoms. Brian feels much better after only a few days.*

Dizziness and balance problems are common symptoms following concussion. Dizziness can be a sense of spinning or a feeling of light-headedness and wooziness. The sensation of spinning is known as **vertigo**. Vertigo is caused by a disturbance of the **vestibular system**. Vestibular disturbances are classified as either **peripheral** (coming from a disturbance of vestibular structures in the inner ear) or **central** (coming from a part of our brain known as the **brainstem**).

The inner ear, shown in Figure 3.2, has a variety of small organs that play a vital role in our ability to understand the position of our bodies within space and sense changes in our position. Our inner ears have two small saclike organs (**utricle** and **saccule**) and three **semicircular**

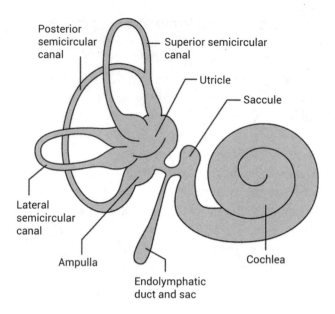

FIGURE 3.2. Diagram of the inner ear

Originally published in Giles Warner, Andrea S. Burgess, Suresh Patel, Pablo Martinez-Devesa, and Rogan Corbridge. Otolaryngology and Head and Neck Surgery. Copyright © 2009, Oxford Publishing Limited. DOI: 10.1093/med/9780199230228.001.0001. Reproduced with permission of Oxford Publishing Limited through PLSclear.

canals that work together to provide information about the orientation of our body and head in space. Small crystals (**otoliths**) within the structures of the inner ear send signals to the brain about the direction of the head. In some cases, the impact of a concussion can dislodge these crystals, which can cause the brain to receive incorrect signals and may produce an unpleasant spinning sensation. If you experience a spinning sensation that is brought on by head movements after a concussion, you may be experiencing a condition called **benign paroxysmal positional vertigo** (**BPPV**). The posterior semi-circular canal (PC) is the most common location involved in BPPV.

If your health care provider suspects that you have BPPV, they may have you quickly change from a sitting position to a lying position while turning your head from side to side to see if this brings on vertigo symptoms. This is known as the Dix-Hallpike maneuver (Figure 3.3).

Your health care provider may also check for causes of dizziness by carefully thrusting your head in different directions to evaluate for abnormal eye movements (called **nystagmus** or **catch-up saccades**) that can occur after a concussion. They may ask you to move your finger from their finger back to your nose several times to check your coordination. To check for balance problems after a concussion, your health care provider may have you walk in a straight line and watch you stand in a variety of different positions. You may also need to try to balance with your eyes closed or while standing on one leg to identify subtle changes in your balance. One test that some providers use to assess for balance problems is called the **Balance Error Scoring System (BESS)**. As part of this evaluation, you will be asked to maintain your balance in three different stances (Figure 3.4) *on both a firm surface (pictures a-c) and a foam surface (pictures d-f)*.

If it is determined that your symptoms are from BPPV, your doctor may try to give you some immediate relief using a procedure called the **Epley maneuver**. The Epley maneuver involves having you lie on your back and hold your head in various positions to help the inner ear crystals (otoliths) return to their correct locations within the ear. If you have BPPV, this procedure can give you tremendous relief.

In cases of vertigo or dizziness that are not caused by BPPV, management may include vestibular therapy to strengthen and adapt your balance and help your vestibular system to recover more quickly. Vestibular therapy is often done by a specially trained physical therapist.

Sleep Disturbance

Concussion can cause a variety of sleep disturbances that make it difficult to get enough good-quality sleep. Following a concussion, you might feel excessively sleepy (a condition called **hypersomnia**) or you might experience difficulty falling or staying asleep, which is called

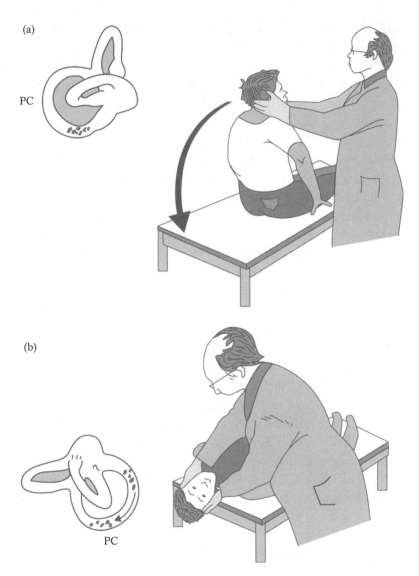

(a)

PC

(b)

PC

FIGURE 3.3. Dix-Hallpike maneuver

Originally published in David Likosky, S. Andrew Josephson, Michael Joseph Pistoria, and William D Freeman. Neurology for the Hospitalist A Practical Approach. Copyright © 2014, Oxford Publishing Limited. DOI: 10.1093/med/9780199969630.001.0001. Reproduced with permission of Oxford Publishing Limited through PLSclear.

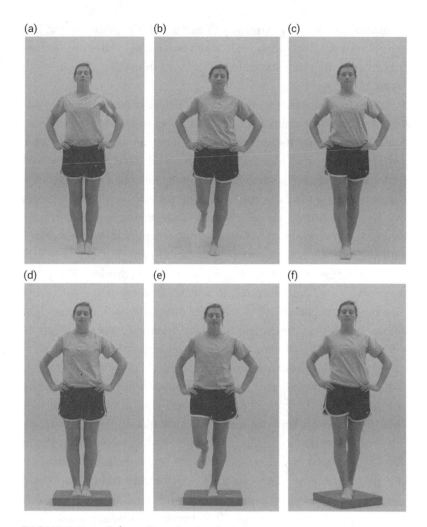

FIGURE 3.4. Balance Error Scoring System

Originally published in David L Brody. Concussion Care Manual, 2nd ed. Copyright © 2019, Oxford Publishing Limited. DOI: 10.1093/med/9780190054793.001.0001. Reproduced with permission of Oxford Publishing Limited through PLSclear.

insomnia. Insomnia is extremely common after concussion and has been shown to affect individuals with concussion even more so than individuals with more severe forms of brain injury (i.e., moderate to severe brain injury).

Other associated sleep problems following concussion that can adversely affect sleep quality include the onset of **restless legs syndrome**, or periodic leg movements during sleep. This can happen if you have a slight deficiency in your body's vitamin and mineral stores. Sleep-disordered breathing has also been observed in some individuals who have sustained a concussion. If your bed partner or roommate hears that you are snoring more loudly than usual or notices pauses in your breathing during sleep after a concussion, it is important to share this with your health care provider. Your health care provider may recommend further evaluation with either an overnight sleep study at a sleep clinic or a home sleep test in which you (or a partner or family member) are taught how to attach some diagnostic equipment at night before bed; this equipment records data about your sleep that can be interpreted later by a doctor who specializes in sleep disorders.

As time progresses, more and more scientific information suggests that good-quality sleep is required to promote the metabolic healing and recovery of the brain following concussion. It is important not only to get enough hours of sleep (adequate quantity) but also to get the appropriate quality of sleep by achieving the deeper sleep stages (**slow-wave sleep**) that are associated with recovery. Insufficient sleep and poor quality of sleep can also contribute to feeling depressed and irritable and can negatively affect your thinking abilities, such as memory and concentration. It is important to discuss difficulty sleeping after a concussion with your health care provider so that they can identify the cause and recommend appropriate treatment.

Although it can be very tempting to use over-the-counter sleep medicines when you are not sleeping well, some medications can cause additional problems after a concussion. For example, many sleep aids available at the drugstore contain diphenhydramine (Benadryl), which can cause grogginess the next day. **Melatonin** may be useful to improve your sleep, but it is important to check any over-the-counter drugs with your doctor to make sure they are okay to use after a concussion. In addition, keeping a consistent sleep schedule, such as going to sleep at the same time every night, is very important. Avoiding use of caffeinated food and drinks after 2 p.m. and avoiding naps will both help you get more restful sleep at night. A "wind-down" routine each night that involves relaxing activities, such as listening to soft music or drinking herbal tea, helps your body get ready for sleep. In the evening before sleep, it is also very important to avoid use of electronic devices that emit light such as smartphones, e-tablets, laptops, and televisions. These devices emit light that can activate or wake up your brain. Some people find it helpful to use an eye mask to block out other light and a fan to block out sounds that might disturb sleep.

When sleep problems persist after a concussion, a variety of possible treatment options can be discussed with your clinician. More information about the treatment of persisting sleep disturbance after concussion is presented in Chapter 7.

Fatigue

One of the most prominent symptoms after concussion is a widespread feeling of fatigue and lack of energy, which affects both physical and mental abilities. Shortly after the concussive injury, you may experience very profound fatigue. Fatigue typically refers to feeling exhausted even after a full night of sleep. You may find that you sleep a great deal more than usual in the first couple of days after a concussion and have reduced energy to complete typical activities. Initially, it is important to have this short period of rest and to get some extra sleep. After a few days, however, it is important to begin walking daily. Gentle exercise can be very helpful in coping with fatigue and regaining energy. Your brain may also seem as though it is tired. This symptom is often experienced as feeling that thinking is sluggish or slowed. The early cognitive symptoms of concussion are discussed in greater detail in Chapter 5.

It is important to discuss symptoms of fatigue that persist for weeks after a concussion with your health care provider and look for other factors that might be contributing to the fatigue. Lack of exercise can make you feel very tired and fatigued. Many well-meaning providers have recommended that patients who have had a concussion should stop all exercise until they are completely symptom-free. Since many people who have never had a concussion have occasional headaches, it may be a very long time before someone is completely symptom-free after a concussion. As a result, some individuals may end up with very long periods of inactivity that contribute to them feeling very tired. The lack of exercise can be particularly problematic for athletes or other physically active people who are used to regular and intense exercise. As was discussed in the sleep disturbance section earlier in this chapter, lack of good-quality sleep is also common after concussion and can result in significant fatigue.

It is important to note that feeling unusually tired for weeks after concussion may be a symptom of **depression**, especially if you do not feel rested after sleeping or wake up very early and cannot get back to sleep. It is important to discuss this with a health care provider because depression is very treatable for most people, and effective treatment of depressive symptoms can result in significantly improved energy. Depression is discussed further in Chapter 4, on the early emotional symptoms of concussion.

Summary

This chapter discussed some of the most common physical symptoms of concussion, including sleep disturbance, headache, fatigue, and balance problems. It also provided information about some of the underlying mechanisms that contribute to these symptoms and how your medical providers may evaluate these symptoms and the types of therapies that they may recommend. Chapters 4 and 5 discuss the emotional symptoms and cognitive symptoms of concussion.

4

Early Emotional Symptoms of Concussion

In this chapter, you will learn:

- How concussion can produce emotional symptoms
- How these symptoms may look different in different people
- Tips for managing these symptoms

For some people, concussions can cause changes in **mood** or **behavior**. Mood refers to an emotional state, such as feeling happy, angry, or sad, whereas changes in behavior refer to differences in the way you act or behave. Many of us are used to experiencing different emotions depending on things that happen throughout our days and the ups and downs that come our way. However, experiencing changes in the way that you feel, behave, or respond to things can be concerning, particularly if you are not sure that you have had a concussion. It can be particularly confusing and frightening if you do not know that a concussion can cause mood changes. This chapter describes some of the most common types of emotional and behavioral symptoms you may experience with a concussion and offers some tips to help you manage these symptoms.

Angela has just finished having dinner with friends one winter night when she slips on black ice and falls, hitting her head against the wall as she goes down. She feels woozy but does not lose consciousness. Her friends are headed to another place for one last glass of wine before the end of the night, so she decides to stay out with them a bit longer. When they arrive at the bar, Angela feels overcome by the urge to cry. She goes to the restroom, where the tears flow from her eyes. She thinks, "Why am I crying?" She honestly does not know. The next morning, Angela wakes up with a terrible headache, which she assumes is because of the wine. Her roommate has made breakfast and left a pile of dishes in the sink. Angela snaps at her roommate for always being so messy and says some things that are particularly hurtful and out of character for her. She leaves the apartment and heads to the grocery store to pick up a few things for the week. While there, she becomes overwhelmed and has a difficult time making simple decisions that she usually could make without hesitation, such as deciding which kind of lettuce to buy. After several more days of feeling this way, Angela becomes discouraged. What is going on with her and why can't she snap herself out of it? Why is she feeling this way?

Irritability

One of the many common types of emotional and behavioral symptoms you may experience is feeling like you have a short fuse. You may be easily angered over relatively minor annoyances that wouldn't usually cause you much concern. This is sometimes referred to as having reduced **frustration tolerance**, or decreased ability to manage frustration. In the case example, Angela behaved out of character when she lashed out at her roommate for leaving dirty dishes in the sink. This is an example of how irritability associated with a concussion can look. Although this symptom can be frustrating to the person who has a concussion, it can be even more difficult for family and friends who may not understand the changes in mood and may respond with their own irritability and anger.

What causes irritability after a concussion? Individuals with concussion may become frustrated more easily because of temporary changes within the brain's ability to regulate emotion (to "put the brakes" on emotions). Just as it can be difficult to process information, it can be difficult to process and manage emotions. This is normal and typical after concussion. Situations that might normally be only mildly annoying can result in significant irritability or angry outbursts. Understanding that this irritability is common and expected, as well as temporary, can be helpful, and providing this information to family members and friends can be very helpful in reducing their own emotional reactions. Trying to identify the source of your frustration while you are recovering from a concussion rather than reacting to the irritable mood can reduce the emotional tension for everyone.

Techniques such as deep breathing and **mindfulness** (focusing on the present moment) can be very effective methods of reducing irritability and anger. It can be very helpful to just pause and take a brief moment; many people find it helpful to close their eyes and breathe in as if smelling a flower and then breathe out as if they are blowing out a candle. This simple exercise helps settle strong emotions. Another strategy that can be helpful is based on the fact that concussion can make it difficult to self-monitor or regulate your own emotional response to triggers. Thus, it is sometimes helpful to pick a code word family members can use if they notice your frustration level is starting to rise, such as "volcano" or "thermometer." If your family notices that you are becoming very irritable and frustrated, they can say the code word, which is your signal to pause and take a deep breath. Using a code word can also be helpful for you to signal to others that you are feeling emotionally overwhelmed. If a code word is used, everyone can take a moment to reset and cool down.

Depression

Another common emotional change after concussion is experiencing feelings of sadness or depressed mood. Given the temporary energy changes that occur in the brain after a concussion, the feelings of depression that occur right after injury are likely due to the brain's energy crisis. After a concussion, you may feel sad or blue, fatigued, less energetic, and more tearful than usual. You may also experience changes in your appetite or sex drive. You and others may not recognize sadness or other depressive symptoms as signs of concussion and may be quick to assume the mood changes are because of some other event or experience.

Concussions can be very disruptive to your typical daily routine, which in itself can bring on symptoms of depression. For those who sustain a concussion from a motor vehicle accident, coping with insurance companies, car repairs, medical appointments, and other frustrations can contribute to depression. Dealing with all those things is very stressful even if you haven't had a concussion! Feeling overwhelmed by such stressors and trying to cope with them while feeling both mentally and physically fatigued can also increase **dysphoria**, or low mood. For athletes, absence from sporting activities and teammates can contribute to depressive symptoms. Elite athletes who train regularly may also experience depressive symptoms if they are not able to exercise as much after concussion as they typically do. When you exercise, your body releases **endorphins**, chemicals that make you feel happy and energized. Elite athletes or individuals who exercise more than once per day may be used to getting higher levels of these endorphins than the average person gets and may experience symptoms of depression if their exercise level is dramatically reduced after a concussion. Depression symptoms after a concussion are usually due to a combination of life stress and **biochemical changes** in the brain. Some people may have an increased risk of depression symptoms, however, because of their **genetics**. If you have family members with depression, you may have an increased risk of depression because you share some biological characteristics with your relatives.

TJ is a rugby athlete who sustained a concussion during a preseason game. Before his injury, he was used to exercising two or three times per day in addition to his scheduled practices. After his concussion, he reports to the athletic trainer for practice and is separated from the rest of his team. He feels excluded and worried about how this will affect his status as a starter on the team. He stops getting invited to hang out with his teammates because he isn't around as much, but TJ thinks his teammates view him as weak. He has a lot of negative thoughts about what others might think of him and he isn't feeling good about himself. His energy level is at an all-time low and he finds it almost impossible to get out of bed in the morning. TJ suffers in silence for a long time but ultimately decides that he should talk to his athletic trainer and tell her how much he is struggling. His athletic trainer arranges for him to be seen by a psychologist. He meets with the psychologist for a few weeks until he feels like himself again.

It is important to know that you can experience emotional changes such as depression after a concussion even if you have never experienced depression before or if you don't have a family history of depression. If you do have a family history of depression, however, or if you have experienced a major depressive episode in the past, you may have greater difficulty with depression after the concussion. It is important to tell your health care provider if you have been previously treated for depression, either with **counseling** or **psychotherapy** or with **antidepressant medication,** or if you have had hospitalizations for psychiatric treatment. These factors might increase your risk for prolonged depression after concussion. If you are being treated for depression that is in remission with current treatments, a concussion may make your depression symptoms worse temporarily. If your symptoms of depression last longer than 2 weeks and interfere with your ability to do your typical daily activities—above and beyond challenges you might have due to the concussion—it is important for you to see a mental health provider.

If you have current thoughts of suicide, it is very important for you to see a mental health provider for evaluation and treatment. It is important to share any history of suicidal thoughts or suicide attempts with your health care provider so that they can help ensure your safety and develop a safety plan as you recover from your concussion. It might be important for you to meet with a **psychiatrist** or **neuropsychiatrist** to be evaluated for use of an antidepressant medication as an important part of your recovery. You might also benefit from talking with a psychologist or from a combination of both psychological therapy and medications. If you experience symptoms of depression after a concussion, it is important to realize that you are not alone and that this does not have to be your new normal. Sometimes people are anxious, fearful, or embarrassed about admitting to these difficult emotions. Talking about feeling depressed with your friends, family, and health care provider may be difficult, but you will feel better when you do and they will know you need extra support. Treatments that are available to help you feel like yourself again are discussed in Chapter 8.

Anxiety

Anxiety is also common after concussion, as the concussion can make it difficult to make decisions and can make you feel more worried or overwhelmed than usual. Other symptoms of anxiety include racing thoughts and feeling tense, on edge, or worried. After a concussion, some people experience **autonomic arousal** (activation of the "fight-or-flight" system that increases heart rate and blood pressure), and they think these symptoms are evidence that their concussion is getting worse. It is important to remember that concussions typically do not get worse after the initial period of injury. When it feels as if concussion symptoms are getting worse, it may be that anxiety is playing a role. Feeling anxious about the symptoms can increase the heart rate and cause feelings of shakiness, lightheadedness, and sweatiness, all of which are symptoms of anxiety.

If you feel overwhelmed or anxious after a concussion, it is important to recognize that these feelings are common. Be patient with yourself and with the recovery process and do not become frustrated if you cannot easily turn off the worries or the racing thoughts. It may be helpful to think about anxiety as a natural part of the recovery process. Remember, concussions cause a lot of new life stress and significantly alter your brain chemistry for a short period of time; as a result, you might experience a variety of new mood symptoms, including anxiety. Actively working on mental and physical strategies to reduce anxiety can improve functioning. Participating in light exercise (after you have gotten approval from your health care provider), deep breathing, and relaxation exercises are all great methods to reduce anxiety. If you have anxiety that persists long after a concussion or you experience worries or other symptoms that make it difficult for you to carry out your daily activities, it is important to discuss this with your health care provider. You may need a referral to see a psychologist or counselor who can teach you additional strategies for anxiety management or work with you to reduce anxiety levels through clinical techniques that have been proven effective by research studies.

Having a history of anxiety before a concussion often contributes to increased anxiety after a concussion. Many studies have found that people who report a history of anxiety are more likely to have a complicated recovery process after concussion. Discussing your anxiety with a concussion specialist or knowledgeable mental health provider can help you understand how anxiety affects the recovery process, reduce your worry, and improve functioning. Being open with health care providers about anxiety is important so they can discuss and determine the most effective treatment options for you. Treatment for persistent anxiety after concussion is discussed in Chapter 8, which is focused on assessment and management of persisting emotional and cognitive symptoms after concussion.

Posttraumatic Stress Disorder

Another mental health condition that can occur in the context of concussion is **posttraumatic stress disorder (PTSD)**. PTSD is linked to some form of traumatic event, such as being in a frightening motor vehicle collision or an assault. People with PTSD may have experienced the event, may have directly witnessed the event happening to someone else, or may have learned of its occurrence to a close family member or friend. Symptoms of PTSD can include vividly remembering the trauma (such as in nightmares or flashbacks), being easily startled and extremely alert or watchful, and avoiding anything that reminds you of the injury. For example, if you are injured in a traumatic car accident, you may find yourself avoiding driving or feeling very fearful when driving.

Mental health and emotional conditions are diagnosed using criteria outlined in a manual used by health care providers called the *Diagnostic and Statistical Manual of Mental Disorders* (*DSM*). According to the current edition of this manual (*DSM-5*), the criteria for a PTSD diagnosis include symptoms of at least 1 month's duration that have a significant impact on social functioning and ability to work. The criteria also require that the symptoms are not due to another medical condition or the toxic effect of drugs or other chemical substances.

The *DSM-5* classification system identifies four symptom clusters that characterize PTSD. The first symptom cluster consists of intrusive symptoms, including distressing memories of the traumatic event, nightmares, and **dissociative experiences** in which the subject appears to be re-experiencing the event (i.e., flashbacks).

The second symptom cluster involves active avoidance of distressing memories of the traumatic event. According to *DSM-5*, at least one form of avoidant behavior must be present to make a diagnosis of PTSD. These behaviors may include avoiding external reminders such as people, places, activities, or objects. For example, someone who was involved in a traumatic motor vehicle collision may avoid driving near the site of the accident.

The third symptom cluster describes disturbed emotional states. This refers to persistent negative thoughts and beliefs, such as feelings of worthlessness, hopelessness, shame, and guilt; a sense of **detachment** in interpersonal relationships (which is also called emotional numbing); and the inability to experience positive emotions (**anhedonia**).

Finally, the fourth symptom cluster consists of changes in physiological arousal and reactivity, including being easily startled or irritable; being easily angered; feeling or acting aggressively; being unusually watchful and on edge; and having difficulty sleeping.

If the symptoms develop shortly after the trauma and persist for at least 3 days but less than 1 month, the appropriate diagnosis is **acute stress disorder**. This acute response is characterized by a prominence of dissociative symptoms, such as **depersonalization** (sensation of being out of body) or an altered experience of the environment. Acute stress disorder and dissociative symptoms occurring in the aftermath of trauma are considered strong predictors for the development of PTSD, and both disorders are classified as stress-related disorders by *DSM-5*. In addition, PTSD may have a delayed onset. The current classification system sets a time point of 6 months after trauma to define delayed-onset PTSD.

Summary

This chapter described some of the most common emotional changes that can occur following a concussion and some helpful tips for managing these symptoms in the early days after a concussion. It is important to remember that emotional and behavioral changes are common after concussion, because of both the injury itself and all the stress that can come along with injury. It is important to discuss emotional changes after a concussion with your health care team, especially if you have a history of a mood disorder. Chapter 5 focuses on cognitive symptoms of concussion, which are symptoms that affect your ability to think and carry out mental tasks.

5

Early Cognitive Symptoms of Concussion

In this chapter, you will learn:

- How concussion can cause changes in your thinking
- Tips for managing these symptoms

After a concussion, most people notice some difficulty with their thinking abilities, which are called **cognitive symptoms**. In fact, one of the major factors that determines whether you have experienced a concussion is a change in thinking skills. For many people, difficulty with thinking is clearly noticeable right away but may improve quickly. For others, difficulty with thinking persists for a longer period and can become quite frustrating and anxiety-provoking. This chapter describes some of the most common cognitive symptoms after concussion and offers some tips for how to manage these symptoms.

Eva is a 59-year-old chemical engineer who ends up with a concussion after a minor car accident while driving home from work. A few days after the accident, Eva is experiencing a mild headache and feels more tired than usual but is otherwise doing okay. She decides that she will go to work on Monday at the water treatment plant, where her job requires a great deal of concentration to ensure that the tests she conducts on public drinking water are accurate. For every three water samples that she tests, someone checks at least one of the samples for accuracy, and she does the same for her coworkers. Her coworker notices that several water

47

> *samples that Eva had cleared were, in fact, contaminated. Eva checks her work and realizes that she has forgotten a critical step in the testing process.*

Attention and Learning/Memory

One of the most common problems people experience after a concussion is difficulty paying attention and concentrating for long periods of time. While the brain is recovering, it can be challenging to focus on everyday conversations, read, or listen to important information. This difficulty may be because of decreased ability to focus or increased distractibility (a tendency for the mind to wander away from the task at hand). For example, you may make errors at your job because you forget to carry out steps that are usually second nature to you. If you check your work later, you will likely see exactly what steps you left out; however, in the moment, you likely skimmed over these steps or skipped them completely.

Difficulty paying attention is one of the reasons people who are recovering from concussion may experience forgetfulness or memory problems. Forgetting what your spouse told you to get at the store, where you parked your car, where you put your keys, and why you went into a specific room in your house are all examples of what might be disrupted attention rather than memory problems. When focusing on your headache pain or worrying about your medical bills, you are less likely to concentrate on what your spouse is saying. You might nod your head and seem to be hearing "orange juice and bananas," but the information just slides across your mind, very similar to the old phrase "in one ear and out the other." Lack of attention is very much like working on a computer document but not saving the document before closing it. Similarly, if you do not focus on information long and hard enough to "save it" into memory, it never gets stored in your memory. This feels like you have a memory problem and can be very frustrating, but it is just a temporary problem with your attention.

The good news is that simple strategies can make a difference and help focus your attention during the recovery period. When carrying out tasks that require sustained focus or concentration, it can be helpful to set a timer or reminder to prompt you to stay on task as well as to circle back and catch any errors that you may have made because of drifting attention. If you need to complete an important series of steps at work or while doing tasks at home, it can help to create a checklist of the relevant steps or to ask a coworker or family member to help you make a checklist.

Memory can be thought of as a filing cabinet with drawers that contain files filled with papers, with individual memories making up the papers in the files. If you put papers in the filing cabinet in random order without any kind of organization, it will take much longer to find a specific paper and will likely be quite frustrating. It will certainly be very inefficient! However, if you put a paper in a folder that is labeled and then file that folder in a drawer labeled with information about what is in that drawer, you will be able to find that paper much more quickly and efficiently. Memory is just like that: the more you organize information you want to remember by creating a context or story, the easier it is to recall the information.

The effort you put into learning new information can make a significant difference in how easy or how difficult it is to remember that information later. While you are recovering from your concussion, some simple strategies can help you focus and remember information. Repeating the thing you want to remember and saying it aloud to yourself several times is a good strategy for remembering that information later. Information that is related, such as a story (rather than a list of unrelated words), may be easier to learn because if attention wanders, the context of the story gives clues to link the information you are trying to learn. Therefore, it can be helpful to associate something that you need to remember with a story or visual scene. For example, if you need to remember the code on a keypad to open a lockbox, you may come up with a song that reminds you of the numbers that you need to press. Or perhaps you might see if the numbers that you press on the keypad make a specific shape or symbol. Alternatively, you may tell yourself a story about the numbers. For example, for the code 38225, you might create a story about three (3) friends who went to the store to buy eight (8) hotdogs for a picnic on the twenty-second (22) of May (5). Perhaps the simplest strategy is to write down the numbers and store them in a safe place, such as on a smartphone or in a notebook, for later reference.

Processing Speed

After a concussion, many people also notice that their thinking feels slowed down. Frequently, people report that they can still figure things out and solve problems, but it takes longer than usual. This is called slowed thinking, or reduced **processing speed**. If you are experiencing slowed thinking, your clinician may recommend that you not drive for a few days after a concussion and certainly not in heavy or fast-moving traffic. Driving is one example of an activity that requires rapid information processing and the ability to make quick decisions. It is best if you do not drive after a concussion until your thinking, and especially your processing speed, improves. People who work with heavy machinery may need a few days off work while they recover because their ability to make quick decisions and react to dangerous situations may be negatively affected.

Slowed processing speed is one of many reasons athletes are kept from returning to **contact sports** after a concussion; they are at increased risk for additional injury because they are not able to make rapid decisions or respond quickly to the actions of others. Similarly, military personnel who have a concussion are often removed from duty and sent to a medical center away from action for a few days after a concussion for their own safety and the safety of those around them. For some people, everyday activities such as reading or doing simple math may take longer, so it might take additional time to complete tasks at home, work, or school. Rest assured that taking longer to complete tasks is very common after concussion and will get much better as you recover. It can also help to let those around you know that you will need a little extra time to finish tasks while you are recovering.

Problem Solving

After a concussion, most people are generally still able to solve problems and figure out how to handle new situations, but a variety of factors can make it challenging. The difficulty with slowed processing speed that we described above can make it harder to solve problems quickly or efficiently. Pain, such as headache pain, may also interfere with problem solving. The severe headache that may follow a concussion can make it difficult to solve problems because the pain is very distracting and exhausting. Most people notice that as their pain lessens, their attention improves, and they can more easily solve problems and handle situations that require thinking on their feet.

It is important to realize that symptoms such as anxiety can also make problem solving more difficult, particularly if a problem causes stress or is overwhelming. Some people who sustain concussions from car accidents or falls may also have other injuries from the accident or fall, such as a broken bone. Injuries that occur along with a concussion can make thinking even more difficult because of the extra pain and stress of dealing with two or more injuries. Be patient and accept that solving problems will be harder for a while but will get better.

When recovering from a concussion, it can feel overwhelming to juggle responsibilities and tasks. One strategy is to first clearly identify what needs to be done and make a list. Once you have identified a list of what needs to be done, then rank them in order from most to least important. Start with and focus on the most important problem and see if you can break it down into small steps. The more you break down a solution into small tasks, the less overwhelming your problems will seem. You can then check things off your list as you work toward solving the problem. This strategy can help you focus on small victories; when you've been struggling, accomplishing small goals is a good feeling. You could also consider separating problems into two categories: those that you can easily solve alone and those that might require help from others or take a longer time to complete while you are recovering. Break down problems into smaller steps and then come up with a plan that works for you.

Language

A common concern after concussion is difficulty finding the right word or getting words out quickly. These symptoms tend to clear up relatively quickly, but until they do, it can feel very embarrassing. Feeling self-conscious can cause anxiety and make it even harder to get words out. It is important to remember that many people may not even notice if you are thinking slowly or your attention appears to be wandering, so try not to let the feeling of self-consciousness get you down or interfere with your recovery. As previously described, one of the primary symptoms of a concussion is confused thinking, so it is not surprising that some people may initially also have trouble with word finding. This symptom, however, generally improves pretty quickly. The best way to manage word-finding problems after a concussion is to use other words to substitute for the word that you need and to try your best not to become frustrated. Many people experience word-finding problems after a night of disrupted sleep or when in pain or distracted, and most people are understanding if you have a hard time finding the right word or take a bit longer to do so. Most of us have occasional difficulty with word finding, so everyone can relate. If you have word-finding problems that persist for a long time after a concussion, your doctor may recommend that you be evaluated for other underlying conditions, such as certain types of **dementia** in older patients. Language problems do not typically persist after a concussion, so it is important to see if these symptoms have another explanation.

Executive Functions

Executive functions are a set of cognitive skills that allow you to plan, organize, and carry out goals and tasks. Much as the executive of a company might make big decisions that affect the entire company— such as where to invest energy and effort (focusing attention) or when to shut down a non-performing company branch (shifting attention)—the executive functions do the same thing for your brain. Executive functions allow us to shift from one task to another and then back again when needed to continue where we left off. Executive functions also play an important role in your ability to attend to and solve complex problems, regulate your behavior and emotions, and remain self-aware. A temporary breakdown in the executive system after concussion can be very distressing because it can make you feel as though you have lost control. Changes in executive functioning skills may be particularly noticeable following a concussion as they tend to be worsened by other concussion symptoms, such as difficulty sleeping, mood disturbance, or pain (such as headache pain). After a period of recovery, however, the executive functions will strengthen and an improved ability to function will become more noticeable. If you have preexisting weaknesses in executive functioning or other thinking abilities because of other health conditions, you may have more difficulty with your thinking after a concussion than other people and you may take a little longer to recover. This is discussed further in Chapters 7 and 8 on persisting symptoms after concussion. Table 5.1 lists tips for managing cognitive symptoms during the recovery period from concussion.

TABLE 5.1 Managing Cognitive Symptoms During Your Recovery

Thinking Ability Affected by Concussion	How to Manage These Symptoms During Recovery
Attention	• Stop, look, and listen.
	• Focus on one thing at a time.
	• Reduce distractions, such as by turning off music or the television while doing other activities.
	• Repeat important information.
	• Make notes in a notebook (write it down).
	• Put important information on a whiteboard in a visible place, such as your kitchen.
	• Use sticky notes in different colors to focus your attention on important information.
Learning and memory	• Repeat information that you want to learn and remember several times. Say the information, write it down, and repeat it.
	• Create a story or visual image of information you want to remember.
	• Have a friend quiz you while you are learning information to make it more interactive.
Processing speed	• Allow extra time to complete tasks.
	• Ask for extra time and extended deadlines at school or work while you are recovering.
	• Take breaks as needed since fatigue can slow thinking even more.
Problem solving	• Make a list of problems or tasks that need to be completed.
	• Put the most important problems at the top of the list.
	• Identify which tasks can be completed easily and which ones might require help.
	• See if you can delay solving the most complicated problems until you feel better, or ask for help.

TABLE 5.1 Continued

Thinking Ability Affected by Concussion	How to Manage These Symptoms During Recovery

Language	• If you have trouble getting words out:
	  • Try to substitute a similar word.
	  • Describe the word.
	  • Demonstrate the word.
	  • Try to laugh about it, as we have all been there.

Executive functions	• Reduce distractions. Avoid multitasking, and do one thing at a time. • If someone is talking to you while you are working on something, either stop what you are doing and focus on the conversation or ask the person talking to wait a few minutes. • Remember to focus your attention using the strategies for paying attention.

Summary

This chapter discussed some of the most common cognitive symptoms of concussion and offered some tips for managing these symptoms. Concussion can temporarily affect your ability to pay attention, learn, and process information quickly and efficiently. It can also affect your ability to communicate effectively and confidently, solve problems, or monitor your behavior. Although a variety of strategies can help manage these symptoms in the short term, finding the right strategy can take some time or trial and error. Fortunately, the cognitive symptoms of concussion are usually short-lived, and most people experience a return to their baseline thinking skills within a matter of weeks to months. If your cognitive symptoms are persisting, however, we will talk about that in Chapter 8.

Setting the Stage for Recovery

In this chapter, you will learn:

- What to expect as you recover from concussion
- About factors that may speed up or slow down the recovery process

Although concussion symptoms can be quite uncomfortable and may significantly interfere with typical daily activities, the good news is that for most people, concussions tend to resolve in a matter of days or weeks and most people do not experience long-lasting associated difficulties. Unfortunately, a lot of misinformation about concussion in the media may have you worried that your concussion symptoms may last forever or that you may never be able to get back to your typical daily activities; this could not be further from the truth. If you have sustained a concussion, you should expect to get better and to get better soon. Some individuals do experience longer recoveries, and a variety of factors that influence concussion recovery are discussed in the next section. Just remember, if you are diagnosed with a concussion, it is essential to maintain a positive outlook about your recovery process. It is important not to assume that just because you have a potential risk factor for a prolonged recovery period, that it will automatically take longer for you to feel like yourself again.

How to Promote a Smooth Recovery

So, what steps can you take to promote your recovery process after a concussion? After you've been evaluated by a health care professional, an appropriate plan can be made for you to gradually return to your activities without overdoing it or putting yourself at increased risk of sustaining a second injury (see Chapter 2 for details on assessing and managing concussions). Recovery involves a progressive return to activities that are paced to avoid increasing your symptoms; however, other factors can also play a role in contributing to your recovery.

Factors that may improve the recovery process include maintaining a healthy diet, getting enough sleep, and engaging in regular physical exercise. Eat well-balanced and healthy meals with plenty of fruits and vegetables and minimize fried and fatty foods. In addition, it is very important to stay well hydrated—drink plenty of water! A concussion can reduce your tolerance for alcohol, so avoid drinking alcoholic beverages during your recovery. As discussed in Chapter 3, good-quality sleep can directly contribute to the brain's recovery, so it is important to work with your health care provider to address any sleep difficulties. Recent studies show that staying active after an injury can help the brain recover more quickly following a concussion; exercise has been shown to stimulate the release of a substance known as **brain-derived neurotrophic factor** (BDNF), which actually helps the brain recover. You should talk to your health care provider about how to incorporate light aerobic exercise into your routine. If you sustained other injuries, such as an orthopedic injury (e.g., a broken leg), in addition to your concussion or if you have a preexisting health condition that may make it more challenging to exercise, a physical therapist can help you find an exercise routine to meet your specific needs. The key point is that exercise of appropriate intensity is important in promoting your recovery. It is important to realize that you may have to start with lower-intensity exercise than you did before the concussion, but even elite athletes need to resume exercise at a lower intensity level.

It is also important to acknowledge that having a concussion can be a stressful experience, particularly if you already have stress in your life from school, caregiving, or your job. It is important to try your best to actively manage your stress, as being stressed out about your concussion can actually make the recovery process more challenging. If stress can be addressed early on after your concussion, the risk of persisting emotional symptoms can be reduced. Strategies for stress reduction include listening to a guided meditation, going on a relaxing walk in nature, and practicing deep-breathing exercises. It is healthy to acknowledge any symptoms you may have rather than try to ignore them. Identifying the symptoms and then doing something positive for yourself will reduce your stress levels and help you feel better overall.

It is also critical not to worry or focus too much on mild concussion symptoms because doing so can actually have a negative impact on recovery. Many of us experience mild headaches, fatigue, or even irritability after a long day. If we let these symptoms dictate what we do, we might not be able to do any of the things that are important to us. Remember, concussion symptoms are uncomfortable, but they will not last forever. If you still notice mild symptoms of concussion months after your injury occurred, it is possible that they may be symptoms you had before your concussion that were not as noticeable.

Research also shows that many individuals experience something called the "good old days bias" after concussion. This refers to the tendency after a concussion to feel that you were symptom-free and did not have any problems before the concussion. Most of us experience occasional headaches or misplace our car keys once in a while. However, research has shown that individuals with concussion have a tendency to report having had fewer of these issues before their injury than individuals in the general population. It is helpful to be aware of this bias because it can interact with aspects of the recovery process.

If you are hoping to get back to a baseline that was never quite as you recall, you may never feel as though you have really recovered, even if, objectively, you are back to your preinjury level of functioning. Being able to recognize this bias can help you stay positively focused on your recovery without the negative impact of unrealistic goals or expectations. If you are concerned that you may be experiencing the good old days bias, you should discuss this with your clinician. Although this is a very common experience, you should not automatically assume that you are experiencing this bias, particularly if you have more severe persisting symptoms after concussion.

If you are experiencing more severe symptoms that are not going away, you should schedule a visit with your health care provider so they can rule out any other medical conditions that may be contributing to your symptoms and make sure that you receive appropriate treatment. Chapters 7 and 8 discuss some of the treatments specifically used for prolonged concussion symptoms.

Factors That May Prolong Recovery

Some factors may also prolong the recovery process. For example, teenagers and young children seem to have a longer recovery period than adults and should always be managed more conservatively. It's important to understand that the developing brain may take longer to recover, and special considerations for children and adolescents with concussion are discussed in Chapter 10. People who are older or who have other health conditions may also have symptoms that last longer (see Chapter 15).

Another predictor of a lengthier recovery period is having more severe symptoms at the time of the concussion. Severe headaches, vomiting, and/or having a seizure may indicate a more significant injury, and thus your symptoms may last longer. Having a history of migraines can make headache symptoms or migraines more likely after an injury and can make the recovery process a bit more complicated. When you are being evaluated for a concussion, your doctor should ask you about history of migraines and might even ask if you have family members who have been diagnosed with migraine headaches. Having a family history of migraines might affect how your migraines are treated.

It is very important to tell your clinician about all medications, vitamins, and supplements you may be taking. A prolonged recovery period could be due to some medication or supplements that can affect sleep, energy level, or even thinking, and your clinician can advise you about these. In addition, some people may use substances such as marijuana products or alcohol to help them manage the stress of a concussion. Medications, over-the-counter vitamins and supplements, alcohol, marijuana, and other drugs have the potential to interfere with a recovery process, so it is important to discuss your use of any of these with your health care provider and follow their guidance.

Some evidence suggests that prominent anxiety or other mood symptoms such as depression can translate to a lengthier recovery period, so it is important to discuss these symptoms with your health care provider. The reason for this is unclear, but feeling down, anxious, and worried about concussion symptoms can make those symptoms feel worse. Be very honest with your health care team about any symptoms you may have, including excessive worrying or feeling down or depressed, because acknowledging and treating these symptoms will play an important role in promoting an optimal recovery.

Having experienced previous concussions may also increase the length of your recovery, but not always. If all previous concussions were identified and well managed with full recovery between each concussion, it is possible that a history of multiple concussions will not lengthen your recovery period from a new concussion. Your doctor may monitor you more closely or manage you more conservatively if you have had prior concussions. If you are an athlete, this may mean that you may be held out of practice and competition longer and that you may need to undergo a more comprehensive evaluation before you are allowed to return to competition.

Sex differences may also play a role in the mechanics of concussion and recovery from concussion, although the research on this topic is mixed. Based on current research, female athletes may be more likely than their male counterparts to sustain a concussion. Many reasons have been proposed for this, including differences in neck strength that might affect the amount of force delivered to the brain. Some have also suggested that females are more likely to report acute and persisting symptoms, and thus it is not their recovery that is different from males but the way they report their symptoms. Research on sex differences in sports concussion—and concussion in general—is an important and ongoing area of investigation.

Hormonal factors have also been studied in concussion recovery in women. Some studies suggest that particular phases of the menstrual cycle may be associated with shorter or longer recovery periods, and whether a woman is taking hormonal contraceptive medication might also affect her concussion symptoms. Overall, the results on sex differences suggest that women have increased risk for concussion compared to men playing similar sports and that adolescent females may have longer recoveries. It should also be noted that men have a higher rate of concussion from causes other than sports (for example, motor vehicle collisions) and a higher risk of sustaining a traumatic brain injury across every age group. Since the findings on sex differences in concussion are not clear, anyone experiencing a concussion should be evaluated and managed individually, regardless of their biological sex. It is clear that more research is needed on both age and sex differences to help us understand how those factors might affect the experience of symptoms and the length of the recovery period.

Summary

You can do many things to set the stage for your recovery from concussion:

- Eat well-balanced and healthy meals with plenty of fruits and vegetables and minimize fried and fatty foods.
- Stay well hydrated with water, and avoid alcoholic beverages.
- Keep a regular sleep schedule and try to get good restful sleep.
- After a couple of days of rest, begin walking and gradually resuming your typical activities.
- Do not isolate yourself or avoid all physical or cognitive activities; the goal is to gradually resume your typical activities.
- Tell your health care provider about any medications and supplements you are taking.
- Maintain a positive attitude and focus on small improvements.

Most concussions resolve without any complications, although having a concussion can be both distressing and disruptive to your typical activities. One of the most important things you can do to promote a smooth recovery is related to your mindset. This can be achieved by understanding and accepting that it is normal to experience symptoms after a concussion for a few weeks, but you should not expect these symptoms to become your new normal. However, if you have symptoms that last longer than a few weeks, you are not alone, and a variety of things might be contributing to your longer recovery process, such as your age or other medical conditions. Chapters 7 and 8 discuss symptoms that may persist after a concussion and how they are treated.

Section 2

What to Do If Your Symptoms
Are Persisting After Concussion

Assessment and Management of Persisting Physical Symptoms After Concussion

In this chapter, you will learn:

- What post-concussion syndrome is
- How persisting physical symptoms after concussion are assessed and treated

The majority of people recover from a concussion quickly, but some individuals with concussion will experience symptoms that are persisting beyond the initial weeks to months after the injury. Many clinicians diagnose these symptoms as **post-concussion syndrome (PCS)**, also known as **post-concussive syndrome** or **post-concussional syndrome**. PCS originally referred to symptoms that persisted for 1 month or more after concussion, but over time some doctors began to diagnose patients with PCS in the emergency department, right after the concussion. This misuse of the diagnostic term has created a lot of confusion. Figure 7.1 illustrates the key features of PCS. Since PCS means someone is not recovering, it does not make sense to assign this label when someone has just been injured. In addition, some health care providers think PCS refers to a psychological condition or to a patient who is not invested in their own recovery. As a result, if you are diagnosed with PCS, you may not get the help you need to assist in your recovery. Recent medical evidence has shown that—much like the acute symptoms of concussion—**persisting symptoms after concussion** may be physical, emotional, or cognitive in nature. Treatment for persisting

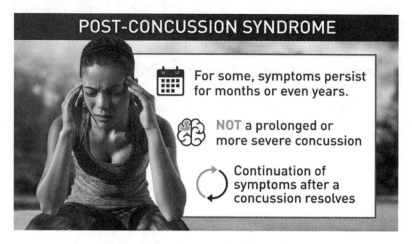

FIGURE 7.1. Postconcussion syndrome
Reprinted with permission from McCarthy MT, Rook R. NeuroBytes: Concussion Versus Post-Concussion Syndrome. © 2019, American Academy of Neurology.

symptoms after concussion can vary depending on the factors contributing to the persisting symptoms and how much these symptoms impair functioning. "Persisting" just means that the symptoms are lasting longer than usual; you may need some extra help to recover, but you will recover! This chapter focuses on persisting physical symptoms after concussion. While we discussed many of the physical symptoms of concussion in Chapter 3, we will discuss how some of these symptoms may be persisting and how they may be treated to help you get back to feeling like yourself.

Assessment of Persisting Physical Symptoms After Concussion

If you had a concussion over 3 months ago and are still experiencing symptoms, you will likely benefit from a comprehensive evaluation to help identify the best course of treatment. It is important to realize that persisting symptoms after concussion can occur for a number of reasons. For example, a headache might be caused by an underlying neck injury, a medication side effect, psychological stress, or lack of sleep. As was explained in earlier chapters, if you are predisposed to a condition such as headache or depression, or previously had one of these conditions, a concussion may trigger or increase the condition and symptoms. In some cases, symptoms can actually become more severe than before the concussion. Symptoms may also be caused by a combination of different factors occurring at the same time.

Cianne is a 19-year-old student at a local community college who sustained a concussion while snowboarding with friends. About a month after the injury, she is still experiencing headaches with sensitivity to light. She wears sunglasses as much as she can and tries to "keep pushing through." She recalls that one of her friends had a concussion and had to do eye exercises. Cianne self-diagnoses her vision symptoms, and because she is having sensitivity in her eyes when she looks up at the light, she assumes that she also needs to do the same eye exercises her friend did. After another month, Cianne is still not feeling like herself. Her headaches seem to be getting worse, and she is starting to feel anxious about not getting better. She decides to schedule an appointment with her primary care doctor, who refers her to an interdisciplinary concussion clinic. Cianne ultimately learns that her eyes are not the cause of her symptoms. Instead, she is experiencing persistent headaches after her concussion, which are making her eyes more sensitive to light. Unfortunately, Cianne's self-diagnosis of her symptoms causes a delay in getting treatment for the true cause of her persisting symptoms.

If your health care provider suspects that you may have persisting symptoms after concussion, they may recommend seeking input

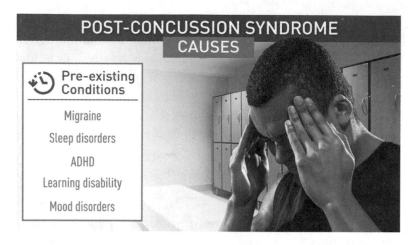

FIGURE 7.2. Preexisting conditions and persisting symptoms following concussion. ADHD, attention-deficit/hyperactivity disorder
Reprinted with permission from McCarthy MT, Rook R. NeuroBytes: Concussion Versus Post-Concussion Syndrome. © 2019, American Academy of Neurology.

from your interdisciplinary care team (see Chapter 2). Some clinics may also provide services in **speech/language pathology** and nutrition. As part of an interdisciplinary assessment, you will be asked to provide information about the event that caused your concussion and to describe what happened around the time of your injury. You will be asked questions regarding details of your current symptoms and your day-to-day functioning, such as the following:

- Are your symptoms improving, staying the same, or getting worse?
- What is your medical history?
- What medications, supplements, or vitamins are you currently taking?
- What is your sleep schedule? Are you sleeping too much or too little?
- What is your current level of activity and exercise?
- What makes your symptoms better or worse?

- Do you have any worries or fears about your concussion?
- What current stresses do you have in your life?
- How are you functioning socially and emotionally? How have you functioned socially and emotionally in the past?
- What is your occupation?
- What is your level of education? Do you have any history of learning problems?

Why are you asked these questions? It is important for care providers to know about your specific symptoms and medical history to create an individualized plan for your recovery. As seen in Figure 7.2, preexisting medical conditions may contribute to symptoms you may experience after concussion. Asking about your sleep, physical activity, and what makes your symptoms better or worse can help the team identify other factors that may be contributing to a lack of improvement. In addition, worries about your recovery, life stress, and emotional distress such as depression or anxiety can all interfere with full recovery. Questions about your occupation, education, and any history of learning difficulties will help the care team understand your level of functioning before concussion so that they can more effectively help you get back to your usual level of functioning at work, school, and home.

Each member of the interdisciplinary care team will conduct an evaluation to best identify the cause of your persisting symptoms; then, ideally, the interdisciplinary team will work together to develop a comprehensive treatment plan to meet your specific needs. The recommended treatment modalities will vary significantly depending on your specific symptoms. For this reason, you should never assume that because a specific treatment worked for someone else it will necessarily work for you. Concussions affect everyone differently, and thus treatment must be tailored to meet your individual needs. Since most people don't see an interdisciplinary team after a concussion, it is important to seek medical attention to address unresolved symptoms rather than assume that someone else's treatment recommendations will work for you.

Treatment of Common Persisting Physical Symptoms

Because you may experience some physical symptoms of concussion that might linger beyond the typical recovery period, we will talk about these symptoms and the importance of getting targeted evaluation and treatment.

Headaches

Headaches that persist for longer than 3 months after a concussion are usually referred to as **chronic posttraumatic headaches**. If you are experiencing persistent post-concussive headaches, a number of treatment options may be suggested by your doctor, depending on the cause of your headaches. Although headaches were discussed in Chapter 3, they are one of the most common symptoms after concussion, so it is important to also discuss them as a persisting symptom.

Anya is driving home from work during rush-hour traffic when she is rear-ended by another vehicle. Her airbag does not deploy, and her head snaps forward and then backward again against the back of the car seat in whiplash motion. Anya does not lose consciousness or experience any changes to her thinking skills but does feel quite startled by what has happened. Her head and neck immediately start to throb. After a few days, her headache and neck pain continue, so she decides to schedule an appointment with her primary care physician to be evaluated. Her primary care physician tells her that she is just experiencing symptoms of concussion and encourages her to rest. However, she continues to have head and neck pain that does not go away. After 4 months of struggling with neck pain and growing frustration that the rest is not helping, she goes back to her primary care physician, who refers her to a concussion specialty clinic. At the specialty clinic, she is evaluated and told that she has recovered from her concussion but has sustained an injury to her neck muscles that is the likely cause of her headache pain. She undergoes physical therapy and is feeling better within a few weeks.

In some cases, it may be determined that your headaches are caused by a musculoskeletal injury to your neck. Neck injuries are a complicating factor in recovering from concussion, particularly when the concussion occurred because of a motor vehicle collision. It is possible you might have had a neck injury and not actually have had a concussion. The diagnosis of concussion requires altered mental status at the time of injury (see Chapter 1). Sometimes individuals do not have any changes in their thinking at the time of an accident, but they have a whiplash injury that affects their neck. Headache pain may develop over the next several days as the neck muscles tighten. The neck pain and resulting headaches can feel rather intense and may disrupt sleep, which can make it more difficult to think, increase irritability, and cause fatigue.

Health care providers may mistakenly attribute symptoms you are experiencing to a concussion instead of the neck injury. Unfortunately, this type of misdiagnosis can delay treatment and result in prolonged symptoms. It is always important to advocate for yourself to make sure your health care provider has conducted a thorough examination. For example, it can be helpful to highlight any symptom that is particularly concerning to you and to ask if referral to a specialist could be helpful. The good news is that most health care providers specializing in concussion and other forms of head injury know how to check for multiple factors contributing to persisting symptoms. This includes considering neck injuries and other underlying conditions that could be making your symptoms worse.

If your health care provider identifies an underlying neck injury, they will discuss different treatment options with you. Your provider will likely want to refer you to a physical therapist who can prescribe neck stretching and range-of-motion exercises to strengthen weak tissue and heal injured tissue, which will reduce your pain level and make you feel much more comfortable. Physical therapists are skilled at treating neck injuries and tightness in neck muscles.

Your health care provider may also recommend that you take a pain reliever/anti-inflammatory medication. You may also receive a prescription for a gel or lotion containing a numbing substance called **lidocaine** to rub on your neck. Lidocaine reduces tightness in your neck muscles and relieves pain. Other options to discuss with your health care provider include **massage** and **dry needling**. Massage can be helpful to loosen muscles in the head and neck and reduce your headache pain. Dry needling is a treatment in which needles (without medicine) are inserted into trigger points in your muscle tissue to release tightness and relieve pain. Many physical therapists are trained in dry needling procedures. In some cases of more severe or persistent cervicogenic headache, your health care provider may recommend **trigger point injections**, an office-based procedure that uses injections of lidocaine into tender muscle areas to help relieve muscle strain. Another procedure that may be used to relieve pain is an **occipital nerve block**, which is an injection of lidocaine (that might be mixed with a steroid) just under the skin in the back of the head to help relieve muscle tension and headaches.

It is possible that your headache pain is caused by chemical changes within the brain as a result of concussion. You may be more susceptible to this type of headache if you have a personal or family history of recurrent headaches or migraines. Although medications can be used occasionally to reduce acute flares of headache pain, when your headaches persist long after a concussion, your health care provider may want to work with you to come up with a daily medication regimen to prevent the onset of headaches. You may be prescribed one daily medication to prevent the onset of headaches (called a **prophylactic medication**) and another medication to use if a breakthrough headache occurs (called a **rescue medication**).

Prophylactic medications work by helping restore balance within the brain's chemistry or rebalancing the part of the brain that triggers headaches, preventing the onset of headaches. These medications can take a while to build up within your system and should be taken every day, even on days when you do not have a headache. In contrast, rescue medications start working right away and are only meant to be taken after the onset of headache or migraine.

Interestingly, most of the medications that are used for headache prophylaxis are approved by the U.S. Food and Drug Administration (FDA) for other uses but have been found to be effective in controlling headaches. These medications include **serotonin-norepinephrine reuptake inhibitors (SNRIs)** and **selective serotonin reuptake inhibitors (SSRIs)**, which were originally developed to treat depressive symptoms but can help prevent the onset of chronic headaches after concussion. Prophylactic medications may also include **antiseizure medications**, such as topiramate or zonisamide, which were developed for control of seizures. Another class of medications used for headache prophylaxis are **antihypertensives** (high blood pressure medicines), such as propranolol or verapamil. Ongoing research is also evaluating newer treatments. In some cases, a medication called memantine, which is used for memory disorders in older adults, may be effective. Some natural supplements have also been shown to help prevent headaches, including daily magnesium and riboflavin.

As we discussed in Chapter 3, a new class of medications called calcitonin gene-related peptide (CGRP) antagonists was recently approved for people with migraine headaches. These larger molecule medications with a long half-life are administered by self-injection once a month as part of a headache prevention regimen. The smaller molecule medications are taken as a pill and are more commonly used as a rescue medication for acute relief of breakthrough headaches. Ongoing studies are evaluating the use of these new medications for posttraumatic or post-concussive headaches.

For people whose headaches do not respond to daily medications after 3 months of treatment and whose headaches occur for 15 or more days a month, injections of **botulinum toxin** (Botox) into the muscles surrounding the head are another treatment option. The FDA recommends a specific procedure for the injections with treatments administered every 3 months. Your doctor may also recommend an FDA approved device that can be incorporated into the management of headaches. These include devices that apply a mild electrical shock to your forehead, upper arm, or neck.

If you are a woman experiencing posttraumatic headaches, it may be helpful to keep track of any patterns that are associated with your menstrual cycle and the onset of headache pain. In some cases, headaches can be caused by hormonal changes within the body and may be effectively managed with contraceptive medications that balance hormone levels.

It is important to stay in communication with your medical team about persisting headaches after concussion and to explore all of your treatment options. Do not lose hope if the first option is not effective. Sometimes it can take a while to identify the most effective medication for you with the least number of undesirable side effects. It is important to limit the number of over-the-counter medications you use as taking these medications on a regular basis can actually worsen headaches.

In many cases, your doctor may also recommend that you work with a psychologist who can teach you behavioral strategies for managing headache pain. Behavioral strategies do not involve medications or medical procedures but usually require weekly or biweekly visits with a psychologist. Scientific research has shown that the following behavioral strategies are particularly effective in reducing pain levels:

- Symptom monitoring and **activity pacing**: this treatment involves tracking pain levels and learning to identify patterns in pain to avoid pain flare-ups.
- **Parasympathetic nervous system** activation: this treatment teaches you to activate your body's built-in relaxation system and reduce pain levels by learning relaxation strategies such as

visual imagery and special breathing techniques. Some specific techniques include:

- o **Biofeedback**: type of treatment that uses sensors that measure muscle tension, heart rate, or skin temperature to provide feedback about the body's response to stress (biological feedback or biofeedback) and how to manage and reduce the stress response.
- o **Progressive Muscle Relaxation**: a guided relaxation technique that involves alternating tension and relaxation of various muscle groups.
- **Mindfulness-based stress reduction** (MBSR) or **mindfulness-based strategies**: initially developed to treat cancer patients with chronic pain, MBSR teaches you how to ground yourself in the present moment, accept the suboptimal situation you may be in, and quiet the mind and its tendency to think about the past or worry about the future. Mindfulness-based strategies have been shown to reduce pain levels as well as symptoms of depression and anxiety, which tend to come along with chronic pain.
- **Cognitive-behavioral therapy** (CBT): this treatment teaches you strategies for identifying negative thoughts and understanding the relationship between thoughts, emotions, and behaviors. Pain can affect your thoughts, feelings, and the way you interact with those around you. If you are experiencing longstanding pain after a concussion, you may benefit from learning CBT strategies that can keep the pain from significantly affecting your quality of life.

Some doctors may only prescribe behavioral pain management strategies if you do not respond well to medication management or dislike taking medications. However, research suggests that these treatments work well when combined with medications. If you experience persisting headache pain after a concussion, you should ask your health care provider about behavioral pain management strategies and psychologists in your area who are experienced in teaching these strategies. It is important to realize that lack of sleep and emotional distress can also make your pain worse. In some cases, your health care team may suggest psychological therapy and/or medications to address these concerns.

Vestibular Symptoms

Some people have vestibular dysfunction as part of their concussion, which may produce dizziness, vertigo, or balance problems. Some concussions cause tiny crystals in the ear to become dislodged and move into another part of the ear (Chapter 3). These crystals tell your brain "which way is up," so to speak. When they become dislodged, you can experience a spinning sensation, as if the room were moving around you. Benign paroxysmal positional vertigo (BPPV) is effectively treated by using simple physical maneuvers that can help get crystals back into their correct place in the inner ear. Sometimes, these symptoms can be treated with a simple manipulation of the head and neck, but occasionally they will take longer to resolve. If this happens, a rehabilitation program administered by a physical therapist (or other vestibular specialist) will be recommended to help you with your recovery.

If your persisting symptoms after concussion include dizziness triggered by moving your head, ask your health care provider for a referral to a specialist in vestibular disorders. A vestibular specialist can work with you to identify the cause of your symptoms using special techniques, such as a **video nystagmogram** (VNG), which uses special goggles with built-in cameras to evaluate eye movements. Additional testing of the vestibular system may be done with either cold water or **temperature caloric testing**, a procedure in which eye movements are measured in response to either cold water or warm air being injected into the ear. These evaluations can help identify whether a problem in the inner ear is contributing to the dizziness. With this information, a treatment plan can be developed to facilitate your recovery.

If your physical symptoms are persisting and do not respond to the treatments discussed, it can be an indicator that some additional complication may be present. Persistent dizziness or lightheadedness that feels worse when standing or after standing for long periods of time may be a sign of **autonomic dysfunction**, which refers to a disruption within the body's system that regulates unconscious functions such as heart rate and blood pressure (our "fight-or-flight" response). Symptoms that get worse with standing or being upright and improve when you are reclining or lying down are called **orthostatic intolerance**. Evidence is growing that concussion and different forms of orthostatic intolerance, including a condition known as **postural tachycardia syndrome** (POTS), may be linked. Many symptoms of POTS overlap with concussion symptoms, including dizziness, headache, fatigue, nausea, visual disturbance, and cognitive symptoms (e.g., mental fogginess). Although the exact relationship between POTS and concussion remains unclear, research suggests that concussion (or physical deconditioning after concussion) may be a trigger for the disorder. The evaluation for POTS usually involves a **tilt-table test**, although other methods for diagnosis are also used. In the tilt-table test, you are secured to a special table and monitored while lying flat and then while the table is tilted up so that you are almost upright. As part of this test, you may also be given medication that makes you feel as if you are exercising and you will be monitored to see how your body responds and what symptoms you have. POTS is usually treatable with lifestyle modifications, such as increasing water and dietary salt intake or, in some cases, with the addition of electrolytes, salt pills, or medication. If you experience persistent dizziness or lightheadedness after a concussion, and especially if you notice that your symptoms get worse when you are standing up, ask your doctor or interdisciplinary concussion team providers about being evaluated for POTS or other forms of orthostatic intolerance.

Persistent fatigue or cognitive symptoms that persist longer than 6 months and do not respond to treatment may indicate an associated problem with your **endocrine system**. The endocrine system is a network of organs and glands that help regulate many systems of the body, including metabolism, energy, blood sugar, blood pressure, and pulse. Dysfunction of the endocrine system is more commonly associated with moderate to severe traumatic brain injury, but an association with concussion has been reported. Although people are most familiar with the thyroid gland, the most common persistent endocrine problems following a brain injury is deficiency in **growth hormone** or **testosterone**. Growth hormone is thought to have a role in human development and recovery following injury. Testosterone deficiency can be associated with fatigue and depression. Identifying these hormone deficiencies requires special testing. Replacement of any deficient hormones is typically managed by an **endocrinologist**, a doctor who specializes in the endocrine system.

Visual Symptoms

After your concussion, you may also experience a variety of changes to your vision, which may further complicate your recovery. Sensitivity to light is a common symptom of concussion, but you may also experience other visual symptoms, such as **convergence insufficiency**. Your eyes work together to focus on objects at different points and distances in your visual field, and this ability can be disrupted after concussion. The eye muscles can become fatigued and less efficient at responding to visual input. Signs that you may be experiencing convergence insufficiency include the following:

- Double vision
- Slowed reading speed
- Words appearing to swim or move around the page when reading text
- Eye discomfort when reading or using a computer screen
- Trouble tracking words when reading
- Difficulty looking up from a page to a computer screen

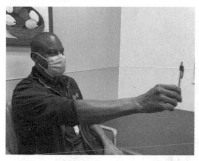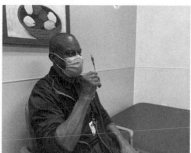

FIGURE 7.3. Pencil pushup

- Visual discomfort, headaches, or feeling lightheaded when trying to read messages on a smartphone

It is important to know that you can have a normal traditional eye examination and still have convergence insufficiency, so a thorough concussion evaluation includes additional maneuvers and examination to measure the near point of convergence, which is how close to your nose a target can be moved before the image becomes double. Fortunately, if you have convergence insufficiency after concussion, you can get symptom relief with some simple exercises. Vision therapy may include exercises that require focusing on moving targets or on a single target, then refocusing your eyes beyond the target. These are known as **pencil pushups** (see Figure 7.3), since a pencil can be used as the visual target. You may also experience relief from eye pain or fatigue through a technique called **palming** (see Figure 7.4). This exercise involves lightly placing the palms of the hands over your eyes for short periods of time to allow the eyes and eye muscles to fully relax.

If you notice particular difficulty with eye fatigue or concussion symptoms that are triggered by visual work such as reading, ask your health care provider to check for signs of convergence insufficiency. Your medical provider may provide you with a referral to a vision therapy specialist who can evaluate and treat any underlying vision problems.

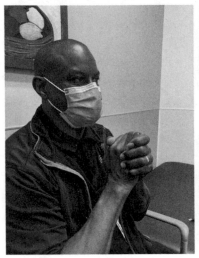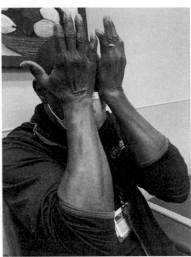

FIGURE 7.4. Palm press

Sleep Disturbance

Sleep disturbance after a concussion is extremely common. One of the most common forms of sleep disturbance following concussion is insomnia, or an inability to fall or stay asleep at night. Sleep problems that linger for months or longer after a concussion can be extremely frustrating and may start to interfere with other aspects of your life. If you are not getting enough sleep, you may feel more emotional, any pain you experience may worsen, and you may have more trouble thinking. Persisting insomnia can make it difficult for you to drive safely or carry out your typical activities at work or at home. If you are struggling with persisting insomnia after a concussion, your health care provider may recommend that you initiate a special sleep therapy called **cognitive-behavioral therapy for insomnia** (CBTi). CBTi works to improve sleep efficiency, which is the amount of time you spend in bed that you are actually asleep. This treatment has three components: improving sleep hygiene, retraining your brain to associate your bed with sleep, and relaxation training.

Sleep hygiene refers to changing behaviors and your sleep environment (your bedroom) to make it more likely that you will fall asleep and stay asleep. Examples of standard sleep hygiene recommendations include the following:

- Avoid caffeinated foods and beverages after 2 p.m.
- Avoid exercise after 3 p.m.
- Avoid taking naps during the day.
- Avoid screen time 2 hours before bedtime.
- Avoid eating large meals right before bed.
- Have a consistent bedtime routine, such as drinking herbal (without caffeine) tea and listening to soft music.
- Go to bed and wake up at the same times every day.
- Use a noise machine or fan in your bedroom to create a monotonous sound that covers random sounds that might awaken you at night.
- Use blackout curtains or a sleep mask to keep light from waking up your brain.

> *Tina is a 58-year-old restaurant owner who has struggled with her sleep ever since she was in a car accident a few months ago. The second she lies in bed, her mind starts racing and she starts to think about challenges at work, her family, the future, and so on. Lately she has found that she can only fall asleep if she lies on her living room couch with the television on. She can usually fall asleep there for at least several hours but never really wakes up feeling rested.*

Temporary insomnia may become more chronic when you start to associate your bedroom and bed with feeling alert. This association becomes problematic because your bedroom is meant to be a place for sleep and feeling sleepy. If you spend many nights awake in your bed after a concussion, your brain may begin to associate your bed-room or bed with feelings of wakefulness. The second component of CBTi involves training the brain to associate the bed with sleepiness again. This process can take up to 2 weeks, and you may find that your sleep may temporarily worsen before it improves. Although it might feel difficult, it is important to follow the recommendations made by your health care provider during this step. These recommendations include using your bed only for sleep or sex and leaving your bed if you are still awake after 15 to 20 minutes. When you leave your bed, you should do something relaxing and only get back into bed once you are feeling sleepy again. If you follow the recommendations of this highly effective treatment, you will start sleeping better.

The final step of CBTi involves relaxation training. Your body has a parasympathetic nervous system known as the "rest and digest system." Learning to activate this system will promote sleep. During this stage of the treatment, you will learn to quiet your mind at bed-time. Learning these relaxation strategies will be very helpful if you tend to do a lot of thinking and planning in bed. Relaxation training may involve learning how to picture yourself in a calm, safe, and relaxing place. Your CBTi therapist (sleep coach) may work with you to write a script you can read to yourself at bedtime or may provide you with audio recordings to help guide you into a more relaxed state. If you have been bothered by difficulty falling or staying asleep, or if you wake up earlier than you would like without being able to fall back asleep, it is best to discuss this with your health care provider, who can help decide if it is time to see a sleep specialist.

Depending on your specific difficulty with sleep, your health care provider may also prescribe medication to help you fall asleep or stay asleep. Whether medications are prescribed for you will depend upon the type of sleep problems you are having and the details of your con-cussion. Most medications are used for a limited period of time, such as 1 to 2 weeks. It is important to know that most medical treatment guidelines do not recommend using prescription medications long term for treating insomnia. If you are having difficulty with falling asleep and staying asleep at the right time (during your usual sleep time), you may be given instructions to increase your exposure to bright light in the morning and limit your light exposure at night as much as possible. Your health care provider may also recommend that you try an over- the-counter supplement called melatonin. When melatonin is taken at the appropriate dose under the supervision of a health care provider, it can help "reset" your body's internal clock. When you reset your internal clock, you will be better able to sleep at night and feel awake and alert during the day.

If you continue to have difficulty with obtaining good-quality sleep after concussion and your health care provider suspects that you may have underlying medical or health issues that are contributing to your sleep problems, you may be referred for a type of sleep study called a **polysomnography** (PSG) study. This study may be done in a sleep center or as a less comprehensive **home sleep test** with special equipment. For an overnight study at a sleep center, you will be given a private room meant to look like a hotel room, and a technician will apply sensors that allow your physician to evaluate breathing, arousals, leg movements, and brain waves during sleep. The home sleep test is a good screen for moderate to severe difficulties in sleep-related breathing, such as **obstructive sleep apnea**. However, the home test does not evaluate brain waves or leg movements. A sleep specialist will review the results of your sleep study and discuss the best plan of action with you. If it is determined that you have a sleep problem such as obstructive sleep apnea or restless legs syndrome, you will receive treatment for the condition and your sleep quality should improve significantly. There is ongoing research to determine the relationship between these conditions and concussion. It is understood that these conditions that affect sleep quality can prolong recovery from concussion if they are untreated. Obstructive sleep apnea is a common condition in which the muscles surrounding the palate or upper airway relax too much and impair the normal exchange of air and breathing during sleep. The key to treatment is, therefore, to keep the airway open during sleep. A number of approaches are available to treat obstructive sleep apnea, but the most common ones involve using a specially fitted dental orthotic or a **continuous positive airway pressure (CPAP)** device. The CPAP device allows you to breathe room air under pressure, which acts as an air splint to keep the upper airway open during sleep. Restless legs syndrome is associated with an urge to move your legs before sleep and can contribute to difficulty in falling asleep. It is typically treated with medication that specifically targets the condition.

Treating sleep disorders can have a remarkable positive effect on your overall physical, emotional, and cognitive functioning. Evaluation of sleep disorders and targeted treatment of insomnia, restless legs syndrome, or obstructive sleep apnea can make a significant difference in your daily functioning and quality of life. When your sleep improves, you will likely feel much better overall.

Summary

Although the majority of individuals with concussion experience resolution of their symptoms after a few weeks to months, this is not the case for everyone. Experiencing physical symptoms after concussion can be extremely frustrating and confusing. You may start to feel discouraged if your concussion symptoms last longer than usual and wonder if this is your new normal. The good news is that many treatments are available if your physical symptoms persist. It is important to discuss your concerns with your health care providers and to remember that persisting symptoms may be the result of a number of factors. It is also important for you to have a new evaluation to look at your specific symptoms and for your health care providers to develop an action plan to treat your individual symptoms. Interdisciplinary assessment is particularly helpful if you have persisting symptoms. Remember, concussion symptoms are treatable. The next chapter discusses persisting cognitive and emotional symptoms after concussion.

Assessment and Management of Persisting Emotional and Cognitive Symptoms After Concussion

In this chapter, you will learn:

- How mood symptoms can complicate your recovery
- Different types of treatment for persisting mood symptoms
- How to manage and cope with cognitive symptoms that persist

Persisting Emotional Symptoms and Management Approaches

It can be surprising to realize that having a concussion can cause mood symptoms, and it can be very frustrating if the mood symptoms persist for longer than you expect. Common persisting emotional symptoms after a concussion include depression, anxiety, irritability, and posttraumatic stress. Concussions can cause disruptions to brain chemistry, and it may take some time to get back in balance. If you experienced significant anxiety or depression before your concussion, you are more likely to have mood symptoms after concussion, and these symptoms might lengthen your recovery period. Even if your anxiety or depression was well managed, it is possible that your mood symptoms might increase after a concussion because of the temporary disruption in brain chemistry. If you have never had clinically significant depression or anxiety, you might develop these mood symptoms after a concussion. In addition to the initial changes in brain chemistry that occur at the time of the concussion, the experience of having a concussion is very stressful, and you might be very worried about your symptoms and how they are affecting your life. You might be having trouble keeping up at work or may be missing school or other important activities. Unlike a sprained ankle that is obvious to others from a compression wrap or brace, crutches, or a limp, concussion is an invisible injury; no one can tell you have had a concussion from looking at you. You may be worried about what others will think if you take time off from work, school, or other activities, or you may feel guilty about taking time off. It can be a very confusing and lonely time, and you may even feel like withdrawing from your friends and family.

If you experience anxiety or depression after your concussion and the feelings do not go away after a few days or worsen, you may benefit from psychological and/or **pharmacological** treatment. Pharmacological approaches often use antidepressants such as selective serotonin reuptake inhibitors (SSRIs) or selective serotonin and norepinephrine reuptake inhibitors (SNRIs) or buspirone. Caution should be advised for a class of medication that has sometimes been used for anxiety that can interfere with recovery. Benzodiazepine medications such as diazepam, or alprazolam, or lorazepam can interfere with brain recovery and may worsen fatigue and cognitive slowness. Your neurologist or health care provider should be informed of any pre-existing medications or conditions you may have to assure a safe and effective regimen is selected if pharmacological treatment will be part of your individualized management plan.

Cognitive-behavioral therapy (CBT) and supportive therapy can be extremely effective in helping you navigate some of the emotional challenges that arise in the context of concussion. CBT (see Chapter 7) helps you identify the relationship between thoughts, feelings, and behaviors and will provide you with skills to catch negative thought patterns and change them into more positive ones. Here's an example of how a CBT therapist might help change a thought pattern:

- Identify your mood: "I feel sad and blue."
- Identify the negative thoughts you had just before your mood changed: "I can't do anything fun now that I have had a concussion."
- Change your thoughts to make them more positive and optimistic: "I need to slow down temporarily, but I'll be back to my usual activities soon."
- Notice the change in your mood from feeling down to feeling more positive.

Your health care provider might also suggest mindfulness-based stress reduction or other mindfulness-based therapies, which have been shown to improve mood, reduce pain, and sharpen thinking skills. These therapies focus on increasing your moment-to-moment awareness of thoughts, bodily sensations, and emotions. Mindfulness can help you live more fully in the moment and be more flexible in responding to your daily challenges. Another important type of treatment for persisting mood symptoms is **behavioral activation**, or an emphasis on getting out and doing things. Your therapist might insist that you engage in one positive activity every day. Examples include meeting a friend for coffee, going on a walk, or planting flowers. Engaging in small positive activities every day can help break the cycle of persisting symptoms of depression after a concussion.

If you feel particularly stressed or anxious after a concussion and your worries last longer than 2 to 4 weeks, your health care provider may also recommend something called **exposure therapy**. Exposure therapy is helpful if you are experiencing both posttraumatic stress and other forms of anxiety, such as fears about going back to work or school or driving. Exposure therapy helps reduce your anxiety and get you back to your preinjury functioning by creating opportunities for you to face your fears gradually and in a safe and supportive environment. For example, if you were injured in motor vehicle collision, your therapist might have you do a relaxation exercise and then picture yourself walking up to your car. Your therapist would then develop a plan for you to work on relaxation followed by increasing your exposure to driving. When you are able to stay relaxed and comfortable thinking about walking up to your car, the next step might be to think about sitting in the car and then driving in your neighborhood at low speeds. Then you might practice staying relaxed while actually sitting in your car, and so on. The goal is to gradually expose yourself to whatever is associated with your anxiety and fears while continuing to practice your relaxation skills. Newer forms of exposure therapy use virtual reality technology to recreate feared situations during treatment. Virtual reality is often used with military service members and others who have posttraumatic stress. In **virtual reality therapy**, you wear large goggles that show a visual image just as if you were really in the situation that caused your fear. The therapist works with you to talk through your fear response and remind you to use anxiety-reduction strategies to manage your emotional reaction. Virtual reality therapy can be very effective because it can simulate the specific triggers of your fear and the therapist can control the duration and intensity of your exposure. An example of **virtual reality goggles** is shown in Figure 8.1. When used for this therapy, the virtual reality goggles are worn by an individual and what they see around them is designed and adjusted by a program managed by the therapy team that can simulate the exact circumstances or situations that are causing the anxiety symptoms and impairment. Before virtual reality goggles were available, exposure therapy used photographs or relied on the imagination of the person being helped, which were not always sufficient. This technology better simulates real situations that may be encountered.

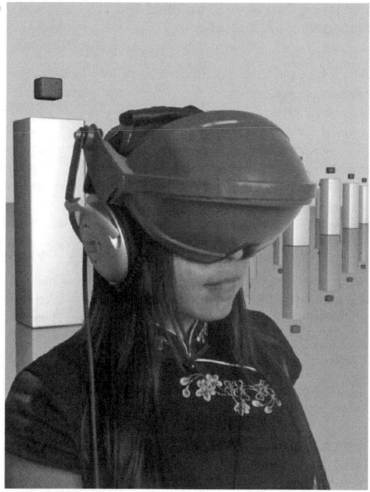
(a)

FIGURE 8.1. Virtual reality apparatus: head-mounted display with embedded motion tracker

Persisting Cognitive Symptoms and Management Approaches

For a few people, disruption in thinking abilities, such as attention, processing speed, executive functioning, and memory, may last longer than is typical. As with any persisting concussion symptom, it is critical that you and your health care provider identify the underlying reason for your thinking problems before starting a program of treatment. Quite often, persisting difficulty with thinking is actually the result of other problematic and persisting symptoms, such as insufficient sleep, headache pain, or mood disturbance. Because persisting thinking difficulties can have so many causes, it is important for you to let your health care provider know about all of the persisting symptoms you experience after your concussion. One particular symptom may be triggering the other symptoms, and that can help inform the best treatment for you. If you need a refresher on these different cognitive abilities, they are reviewed in Chapter 5.

If you were prescribed an extended period of "brain rest" following your concussion, you may also be experiencing mild **cognitive deconditioning** (sometimes called "unplugged syndrome"). This deconditioning can cause temporary slowing and inefficiency of your thinking abilities. This is similar to what happens to your body when you go for days or weeks without physical exercise. Just as your body feels sluggish and you have less energy, your brain can feel sluggish too. If your health care provider suspects that your symptoms are a result of cognitive deconditioning, they will recommend that you get back to using your brain as much as possible in day-to-day life. Your neuropsychologist or other treating provider may also recommend that you participate in special thinking games on a computer or tablet to track your progress as you get back into the habit of exercising your brain. If your thinking difficulties persist months after a concussion, you may be afraid to participate in activities that require focused thinking, especially if the activities make your headaches worse or if you feel a bit more tired. It is important to know that using your brain won't hurt you and will actually help your recovery. In fact, using your brain is critical to get your thinking skills back up to speed.

In some interdisciplinary clinics, you might have a cognitive screening with a neuropsychologist to evaluate persisting symptoms after concussion. A cognitive screening usually takes about 30 to 45 minutes and may be done on a computer or using pencil and paper. You may be asked to complete a variety of tasks that briefly assess your reaction time, ability to remember things, and responses to questions. If your treatment team conducts a cognitive screening and believes you are experiencing cognitive difficulties that are not due to other persisting symptoms after concussion or cognitive deconditioning, a comprehensive neuropsychological evaluation may be recommended to identify other factors that may be affecting your thinking skills.

A neuropsychological evaluation may take 3 to 4 hours or some-times longer, so it is important to take snacks or anything else that will help you stay comfortable throughout the day. The neuropsychologist may work with a technician who will administer standardized tests of a variety of different thinking abilities, including attention, learning and memory, problem solving, and speed of information processing. In addi-tion, you may be asked to draw geometric figures or identify patterns as part of the evaluation. Neuropsychological assessments are helpful for understanding your strengths and weaknesses and can help identify un-derlying issues that could explain why you may have persisting cognitive symptoms after concussion. In many cases, another medical or neuro-logic condition that did not become noticeable until after the concus-sion may be causing the symptoms. Figure 8.2 shows other causes for symptoms that are persisting after a concussion; identifying and treating or managing each individual symptom is key to recovery.

After the evaluation, the neuropsychologist will provide you with in-formation about your results. You will learn your specific strengths and weaknesses and receive recommendations or strategies to help your per-formance at work, school, or home while you are recovering. The neuro-psychologist will also provide an expert interpretation of other factors,

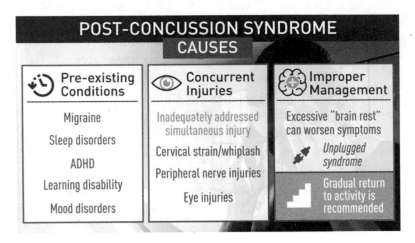

FIGURE 8.2. Factors associated with persisting symptoms following concussion. ADHD, attention-deficit/hyperactivity disorder
Reprinted with permission from McCarthy MT, Rook R. NeuroBytes: Concussion Versus Post-Concussion Syndrome. © 2019, American Academy of Neurology.

such as sleep disturbance or mood concerns that may be affecting your thinking. Although a concussion does not typically result in long-lasting cognitive changes, concussions can make it temporarily difficult to perform at your best. You may need to use strategies to help compensate for the temporary disruption in your thinking abilities.

If the neuropsychological evaluation shows that you are experiencing difficulties with aspects of attention, your neurologist, neuropsychologist, or occupational therapist may help you learn strategies for increasing your awareness in the present moment and for reducing distractions. Staying organized, making concrete goals, setting timers, and getting enough sleep at night can all improve attentional skills. Your neurologist or other health care provider may also prescribe a **stimulant medication**, such as methylphenidate (Ritalin) or dextroamphetamine-amphetamine combinations (Adderall), to stimulate the parts of your brain responsible for maintaining focus and attention. If you are prescribed stimulant medication for treatment of inattention, you may need to be monitored closely for potential side effects, such as reduced appetite and sleep disturbance. Your neurologist or other health care provider may ask you to see a psychiatrist, who will manage this medication for you and will check up on you every 3 to 4 weeks.

Persistent difficulties in memory, especially in older individuals, may be an indicator that an underlying and pre-existing memory problem became more noticeable or possibly worsened due to the concussion. If a pre-existing memory disorder is suspected, some neurologists and health care providers may choose to treat you with a medication known as a **cholinesterase inhibitor** to specifically target memory function. Some examples of these medications include donepezil and rivastigmine and galantamine. Memantine, is another medication that has been used to reduce memory decline, primarily in older adults with significant cognitive decline. In the setting of concussion, it has been used as a preventive medication for headache control. In some cases, memantine may be selected if an individual has both headaches and cognitive dysfunction. It is chemically related to a medication called amantadine which is used in moderate to severe TBI. Studies on the efficacy of amantadine for these persisting symptoms after concussion have had mixed results.

If you experience persisting difficulties in attention, planning, organizing, or memory, your neuropsychologist may recommend that you participate in computerized interventions designed to help you improve in these areas. These computer programs usually involve weekly sessions with a rehabilitation specialist with homework assignments between visits. The rehabilitation specialist may also encourage you to use **compensatory strategies** to help you adjust to any prolonged cognitive difficulties. There are a variety of professionals who may be helping you with cognitive training and compensatory strategies. These include neuropsychologists, rehabilitation psychologists, occupational therapists, and speech/language pathologists. Examples of compensatory strategies include the following:

- Setting aside some time each week to plan ahead for the tasks you will need to complete and prioritizing which tasks are most important
- Entering appointments in your smartphone calendar or on a paper calendar
- Setting an alarm on your smartphone or watch to remind you of appointments, meetings, or other important commitments
- Putting sticky notes on your front door, on your computer, or in other visible locations to remind you of important information
- Repeating work assignments back to your employer or coworker and then writing them down
- Reducing distractions in your environment and limiting multitasking, including turning off the television and music while you are working
- Doing your most important tasks during the time of day when you feel most alert

Compensatory strategies are just simple methods to create structure and reminders while you are recovering—it's like having an external brain!

Summary

This chapter discussed persisting cognitive and mood symptoms, which can be quite frustrating and challenging. Psychological conditions, such as depression and anxiety, are treatable, and getting appropriate treatment can significantly improve your day-to-day functioning. Persisting difficulties with thinking after concussion are often caused by insufficient sleep, pain, or mood symptoms. Getting a good evaluation can be helpful to identify the cause of your particular difficulties, develop a specific plan of treatment to help you feel better, and provide you with strategies for managing your daily activities.

Later Complications

Chronic Traumatic Encephalopathy and Neurodegenerative Conditions

In this chapter, you will learn:

- What chronic traumatic encephalopathy (CTE) is and how it is different from persisting symptoms after concussion
- That the symptoms attributed to CTE and other neurodegenerative conditions may be due to other treatable causes and require a thorough clinical evaluation for accurate diagnosis and treatment recommendations

There have been studies describing a connection between head injuries and an increased risk of developing a neurodegenerative condition later in life in a small percentage of people. This is different than persisting symptoms after concussion. These neurodegenerative conditions present many years after injury and have a progressive worsening course as opposed to persisting symptoms following concussion which occur after the injury but generally do not get worse. The association between frequent recurring concussions and sustained exposure to impact forces and later-life neurologic symptoms is an important and evolving area of understanding.

Chronic Traumatic Encephalopathy

In recent years, a small number of retired professional athletes who have been diagnosed with dementia or suspected to have a type of neurodegenerative process called **chronic traumatic encephalopathy (CTE)** have received prominent media attention. CTE has been associated with playing sports in which athletes experience many impacts over multiple years.

CTE refers to a specific type of pathology within the brain that currently can only be diagnosed by doing a brain autopsy after the affected person has died. CTE falls into a group of disorders known as **tauopathies**, meaning that a primary characteristic of the disease is thought to be a problematic buildup of a protein in the brain known as **tau**. In a normally functioning brain, tau serves the essential role of stabilizing the structural supports of **neurons**, known as **microtubules**. Within the cells of the brain (neurons), microtubules can be thought of as railroad tracks that provide structure for the cells, whereas tau serves the function of railroad ties, helping to bind together these supports for the cells. In certain disease states, tau protein can break away from the microtubules, fold up, stick together, and accumulate within the brain, causing abnormal folding of the structural support of cells. Some scientists believe that in CTE, repeated head impacts over time increase the likelihood of tau protein detaching from microtubules, thus increasing the associated brain changes. Many questions remain unanswered, however, including why this process does not occur for everyone who experiences repetitive head impacts.

It is understandable that you may be worried that you have CTE if you have persisting symptoms after concussion because stories in the press make it seem as if many, or even most, athletes will develop CTE. Unfortunately, at this time, CTE can only be diagnosed at autopsy after a person has died and the individual or their family has donated their brain for autopsy. Our understanding of the true number of athletes or others who might have CTE is limited because so many athletes and those exposed to numerous injuries over years do not donate their brains, especially if they are not experiencing any symptoms. Because we do not have information from brain autopsies of a larger selection of athletes, we do not have a good understanding of what percentage of people who have had repeated concussions actually develop CTE. We need more information from those who have been exposed to repeated concussions or impacts to the head and who have not developed symptoms suggestive of CTE—that is an important priority for future research. This will help us understand why some people may develop CTE, whereas others do not.

It is important to realize that most people who experience a single concussion, which is a temporary neurologic state, do not have any lasting cognitive, emotional, or physical symptoms. If you have a single concussion or even several concussions, it is very different from repeated chronic forces to the brain from concussions and **subconcussive injuries** occurring over many years. Although the majority of people recover from a concussion, you may be one of those who have persisting symptoms after concussion. We discussed evaluation and treatment for persisting symptoms after concussion in Chapters 7 and 8. Evaluating persisting symptoms after concussion in living individuals is very different from diagnosing CTE by brain autopsy in those who had a long clinical history of progressive decline and continued worsening of symptoms. For those found to have evidence of CTE at autopsy, the clinical history typically shows that the progressive symptoms often began many years after their exposure to repeated injuries and continued to worsen after onset. This is a very different history than in those with persisting symptoms after concussion who do not have a progressive decline but become frustrated by their lack of recovery.

Subconcussive Injury

More recently, concern has been raised about subconcussive injury and the long-term effects on health. Subconcussive injury is generally thought to be a type of chronic injury in which repeated impacts to the brain affect the brain's functioning but are not of sufficient intensity to result in symptoms that are noticeable to you or that can be observed by others. For example, many athletes take repeated hard hits to their heads or bodies throughout a professional career. Unlike a concussion, which causes symptoms that are observable and ideally identified and diagnosed, this more subtle type of brain dysfunction isn't detected. Therefore, athletes continue to play without realizing the potential for damage that could be caused by repeated impacts. Scientists are trying to gain a greater understanding of how these forces might affect brain health over the long term. Subconcussive injury is of greater concern in high-impact sports, such as American football, in which athletes are often exposed to multiple hits during games or full-contact practices.

Sophisticated research imaging technology has been used to take detailed pictures of the brains of athletes in contact sports before their sport season begins. Athletes who have not had a documented clinical concussion then undergo the same brain imaging at the end of the season. Evidence of the effects of repeated exposure to subconcussive injuries has been seen in some of these sophisticated research-based brain imaging studies, suggesting that repeated forces to the head that are not sufficient to cause an observable concussion may still be causing some changes in the brain. It is not clear whether these changes are temporary (and resolve during the off-season) or can accumulate and persist over time. For those individuals found to have CTE at autopsy, it is understood that exposure over many years to concussions and chronic impacts were an important contributory risk factor to their development of CTE.

Some recent studies have identified the type of specific training drills in practice that may expose players to subconcussive injuries, and the selection of drills has been adapted by various sports organizations and modified to reduce the overall exposure to forces that might cause subconcussive injury. Many amateur, collegiate, and professional sports teams now minimize the number of practices with drills that involve collisions with another player (such as tackling drills) or with an object (such as football blocking sleds) with the goal of increasing player safety.

Diagnostic Challenges in CTE

Researchers are actively trying to understand what types of symptoms and difficulties individuals with CTE pathology might have experienced before their death. The term **traumatic encephalopathy syndrome** (TES) has been used to describe the collection of symptoms and diagnostic findings someone with CTE may have before death. There are suggested research criteria for TES, but there are not yet validated clinical criteria for this syndrome. A challenge for clinicians is that many of the symptoms attributed to TES/CTE are not specific to these diagnoses. That means that some of these symptoms, including changes in thinking such as decreased memory and attention, mood changes such as irritability and depression, and unusual behaviors, could have other causes. Some have also been reported to have had abnormal motor symptoms such as tremors. Cumulative exposure to concussions or subconcussive injuries and long-term complications such as cognitive decline or mood disorder may be connected in ways not directly related to the tau pathology found in CTE. Symptoms affecting memory, mood, and behavior are commonly found in a variety of other health conditions as well as in the minority of patients who have persisting symptoms after concussion.

Unfortunately, publicly available information does not always explain the uncertainty about the actual **prevalence** among those who have exposure to repeated injuries. The increased awareness of CTE may make you fearful, anxious, and worried. Your family and loved ones may be worried, too, especially if you currently play or have played contact sports. If you are concerned that you may have TES/CTE, it is important for you to talk with your health care provider and ask to be referred for an interdisciplinary evaluation to identify or rule out other conditions that could be causing your symptoms. Understanding the cause of your symptoms is especially important because many health conditions have symptoms similar to TES/CTE. To date, no treatment specific to CTE has been identified. However, treatments are available for some of the other conditions that can cause symptoms similar to those reported in people later found to have had CTE at autopsy. These treatments can significantly reduce the severity of symptoms and improve both function and quality of life. This is an important reason why careful and accurate clinical evaluation of your symptoms is so important: It is critical to identify symptoms that have another cause and can be treated.

Some athletes become so concerned about CTE that they become extremely worried or depressed. Depression and anxiety triggered by the fear of CTE can become debilitating and may even affect thinking abilities. When anyone is very depressed or anxious, everyday problems can feel overwhelming, and it can be hard to engage in day-to-day activities. Athletes then start to worry that these mood-related symptoms are evidence of CTE, further increasing their fear and worry and compounding their psychological distress. Symptoms of clinical depression include slowed thinking, reduced ability to concentrate, and impairment in daily functioning. Mood symptoms can be effectively treated, so it is important not to assume that symptoms in athletes are due to CTE and untreatable.

Continuing research on the mechanisms of CTE and the development of techniques and criteria for the diagnosis of CTE before death (TES) can help us learn more about the earlier changes that begin a pathway of degeneration leading to tau accumulation in the brain. Some researchers have studied the use of advanced imaging techniques that can identify accumulations of tau in the brain. These techniques have proven to be valuable for accurately identifying Alzheimer's disease pathology in patients while alive, but there has not been the same success with other forms of tauopathies like CTE. This is an active area of research. Because of the lack of consistency in these studies, the FDA has specifically stated that current tau imaging is not approved for the diagnosis of CTE. Our understanding of traumatic encephalopathy syndrome is currently limited, but additional research could lead to the development of specific treatment options. Further research is also needed to identify the factors that make some people more vulnerable to TES and CTE than others so that prevention efforts can be refined and improved and athletes can make informed decisions about participating in contact sports considering their personal safety risk.

Neurodegenerative Conditions

Research indicates that people who sustain a moderate-severe traumatic brain injury may have an increased risk of onset of Alzheimer's dementia at an earlier age than the average population. Researchers believe there may be some genetic factors that contribute to the development of Alzheimer's dementia in these people. One example is that the genetic finding of a gene called Apo e4 is associated with an increased risk of Alzheimer's dementia in those without any history of head injury and that the presence of Apo e4 has also been associated with a more prolonged recovery following head injury. Research is ongoing into the relationship between head injury, including milder injuries such as concussion, and later life risk of Alzheimer's dementia.

Studies have described a potential link between traumatic brain injury of all severities, including concussion, and **Parkinson's disease**. This is a disease associated with resting tremors, rigidity, slow movements, and difficulty with balance. Parkinson's patients who reported a past history of head injury were found to have been diagnosed with Parkinson's disease two years earlier than those without a head injury history. Moderate-severe TBI has also been associated with an increased risk of **amyotrophic lateral sclerosis** (ALS). This is a condition associated with progressive weakness of arms and legs, as well as muscles used for talking and swallowing. There is no consensus on whether there is any association between a single concussions and ALS. There are some reports of frequent recurrent concussions being associated with ALS. As with other neurodegeneration syndromes, those who develop either Parkinson's disease or ALS are also thought to have some genetic contribution to the development of these conditions.

Research in this area is helping us understand the relationship between certain genetic factors and head injuries that might lead to the later development of neurodegenerative conditions. One theory is that head trauma may trigger brain changes such as an accumulation of abnormal proteins that may eventually lead to the development of neurodegeneration.

Summary

Hearing stories about former athletes diagnosed with neurodegen-erative conditions such as CTE at autopsy is both sad and anxiety-provoking. Any athlete who is worried or concerned about the cumulative effects of multiple concussions, exposure to subconcussive injury, or CTE or any neurodegenerative condition should ask their health care provider for a multidisciplinary referral to include neuro-logic and neuropsychological evaluation. It is important to remember that regardless of the cause of your symptoms, health care providers can help you feel better and better manage your symptoms. You may experience persisting symptoms after concussion, or you may have other medical or neurologic conditions that are treatable. To better understand your symptoms, a thorough evaluation and accurate diagnosis are critically important. As discussed above, evaluating and diagnosing mood and cognitive symptoms is important so that you can be referred for appropriate evaluation and treatment. Many different factors can affect both mood and memory, and evaluation by knowledgeable health care providers can sort these out. Please do not suffer in silence and just accept your situation. Ask for help. Receiving appropriate evaluations and effective treatments for your specific symptoms will significantly improve your daily functioning and quality of life.

Section 3

Special Considerations

10

Concussions in School-Age Children and Adolescents

In this chapter, you will learn:

- How concussion symptoms may look different in children
- How pediatric concussions are evaluated and managed
- Considerations for return to learning
- General academic adjustments that can be made for the student with a concussion
- Academic adjustments that can be made for students with specific concussion symptoms
- Considerations for the college student with concussion

Children and adolescents are at increased risk of getting concussions, and research has shown that they may also take longer to recover. If you suspect your child has sustained a concussion, it is important that you closely monitor your child's behavior and mood and discuss any relevant changes with your child's pediatrician or other health care provider. Careful questioning and observation by the health care provider and information obtained from you or other family members can be helpful in identifying symptoms. Concussions can be more difficult to identify in children who do not have the communication skills to describe their symptoms. Young children in particular may have difficulty verbalizing their symptoms or may have limited awareness of specific symptoms; they may use general terms, such as stating that they feel "bad" or "sick." Young children may also seem to act out or become more easily frustrated after a concussion.

> *Ty is playing in the living room when he trips on one of his toys and hits his head against the coffee table. His mother does not see him hit his head and does not know he is injured. He continues to play after a short break but seems irritable for the rest of the night and says that he does not feel well. The following day, his kindergarten teacher notices that he is behaving differently; he is throwing tantrums, lashing out at other children, and refusing to eat during snack time. Hearing this, his mother decides to set up an appointment with his pediatrician to see if he has an ear infection or other illness that could explain his behavioral changes. After evaluating Ty and finding a "goose egg" on his head and subsequently gathering additional relevant historical information, the pediatrician diagnoses Ty with a concussion.*

Although adolescents have typically developed communication skills that enable them to convey their symptoms to their families and health care providers more clearly, adolescents with concussion may be more likely than younger kids to isolate themselves from their peers or to experience guilt or self-blame. If you notice changes in your child's or adolescent's behavior or mood, be sure they are evaluated by a health care professional who has expertise in working with kids. Clinicians who have training in pediatrics and work with children regularly are in the best position to identify symptoms of concussion in a child and provide the appropriate recommendations. A number of guidelines have been established to help clinicians provide the best care possible to children and adolescents with concussion and are described below.

Evaluation and Management Guidelines for Pediatric Concussion

The U.S. Centers for Disease Control and Prevention (CDC) convened a group of experts in pediatric concussion to establish guidelines on the diagnosis and management of concussion, which were published in 2018. These evidence-based guidelines are based on an extensive review of published scientific research. These recommendations and resources for parents and schools are freely available on the CDC website (*cdc.gov/HEADSUP*). If your health care provider suspects that your child may have experienced a concussion, you can expect that they will follow the recommendations from the CDC workgroup, including:

- Initial evaluation
  - Evaluating to rule out more severe injury or other injuries or symptoms also needing treatment (e.g., broken arm, trouble with vision)
  - Identifying any other factors, such as dehydration, that might be contributing to your child's symptoms
  - Avoiding CT or MRI scans unless there are specific clinical symptoms that need further evaluation with head/brain imaging (Box 10.1) to avoid exposing your child to unnecessary radiation
  - Using validated and well-researched clinical measures to evaluate symptoms
  - Identifying risk factors associated with poorer outcome (Box 10.2)
- Follow up with your child's doctor immediately if they have any of the following symptoms:
  - Worsening headache that does not go away
  - Repeated vomiting or severe nausea
  - Agitation, restlessness, or worsening confusion

BOX 10.1 Guidelines for the Use of Neuroimaging After Mild Traumatic Brain Injury (Concussion)

- Child under 2 years old
- Continued episodes of vomiting
- Loss of consciousness
- Method of injury was severe
- Headache that is severe or worsening
- Loss of memory
- Scalp hematoma (localized swelling filled with blood) not on the forehead/frontal area
- Glasgow Coma Scale score less than 15
- Clinician suspects a skull fracture

Source: *cdc.gov/traumaticbraininjury/PediatricmTBIGuideline.html*

  o Unusual drowsiness, difficulty waking up, or slurred speech
  o Decreased coordination, increasing weakness, or numbness
  o Seizures, convulsions, or loss of consciousness
- Management of your child's concussion and recovery after concussion
  o Have your child rest right after the concussion and take it easy for a few days (usually 2 to 3 days).
    - Limit activities so symptoms don't worsen. In some situations, the use of electronic devices and video games may worsen headaches or vision or eye discomfort; this may require limiting their use during recovery.
    - Encourage good-quality sleep at night and naps as needed. Note that the recommended number of hours of sleep for children and teens for optimal function is greater than the recommended amount for adults.

BOX 10.2 **Factors Linked to Poorer Outcome After Concussion**

- Older children/adolescents
- Hispanic ethnicity*
- Lower socioeconomic status
- Previous intracranial brain injury
- History of mild traumatic brain injury or increased symptoms before the current injury
- Psychiatric or neurologic disorder
- Lower cognitive ability or learning difficulties
- Social and family stress

---

*This may be because of reduced access to resources or some other social or cultural factors and may not be related to genetic or inherited factors. More research is needed for us to understand this research finding.

Source: *cdc.gov/traumaticbraininjury/PediatricmTBIGuideline.html*

- Provide relaxing activities, such as playing with toys or drawing.
- Demonstrate a positive attitude and help your child feel positive.
o Within a few days and as your child begins to feel better, encourage gradual return to activities.
- If an activity worsens symptoms, temporarily cut back on that activity.
- Encourage short walks outside.
- Emphasize maximum sleep at night.
- Reduce naps or return to regular napping schedule (for younger children).

- Ask your child's doctor about medicine that might help symptoms—for example, headache medicine such as acetaminophen or ibuprofen.
- Limit caffeinated beverages and food to optimize your child's sleep.
  - Encourage your child to resume most activities, including a regular school schedule, when symptoms are nearly gone.
    - Have them take breaks if symptoms worsen.
    - Encourage outdoor play, such as walking and playground time.
  - Support your child in getting back to regular activities other than sports.
    - Your child has recovered when regular activities do not cause concussion symptoms.
    - If symptoms return, contact your child's doctor.
    - With approval from the doctor, your child is now ready to begin the process of return to sports if they are participating in athletics; ask for written clearance and written instructions to share with the coach or athletic trainer.
    - Your child should never return to sports on the same day the concussion occurred. Chapter 12 provides more information on sports-related concussions and the return-to-sport process.

The above recommendations are important guidelines to keep in mind as you seek medical evaluation for your child with a possible concussion and as you monitor your child after a concussion has been diagnosed. Remember, it is always important to have your child evaluated if you believe they may have a concussion. To ensure that your child receives the best care, you might consider asking your child's health care provider if they follow the CDC guidelines for concussion management or if they have any other specific recommendations for your child.

Return to Learning

One of the biggest challenges for children and adolescents is participating in school and educational activities while recovering. The cognitive symptoms of concussion, such as difficulty paying attention and slowed thinking, can make it difficult to learn and keep up with classroom and homework assignments. For high school students who may be worried about grades and college applications, keeping up with schoolwork can become a major worry, and the associated stress and anxiety can complicate recovery. Visual symptoms can also affect school performance, particularly since so many schools now use computers, electronic tablets, and electronic whiteboards. For someone recovering from concussion, looking at a computer screen can trigger headaches, dizziness, or feelings of nausea or lightheadedness. The loud sounds of classrooms, changing classes, and walking through crowded hallways can also trigger symptoms, particularly early in the recovery process.

Right after a concussion when the symptoms are most severe, many students may require 1 or more days of complete absence from school. Students with persisting headaches, difficulty with vision or hearing, and disrupted thinking skills are most likely to have challenges in the learning environment. Identifying a specific staff member within the school to help the student navigate their recovery and facilitate communication with teachers once they return to school is critical. The key staff member may vary across different school systems, so it is important to contact the school and find out who fills this important role. Some schools may have a **school psychologist** or neuropsychologist who can facilitate communication between teachers and parents and help your child navigate the return-to-learn process. In other schools, a school nurse or guidance counselor may play the important role of advocating for your child. If your child is injured through involvement in a sport or is a student-athlete, the athletic trainer may be in the best position to monitor your child's symptoms, communicate with their teachers, and assist in guiding the return-to-learn process.

If your child does not have an athletic trainer, be sure to ask your child's health care provider to make recommendations for school. Detailed resources for school accommodations are available on the CDC website.

An important principle of concussion management in children and adolescents is that return to learn should always occur before return to sports. If your child cannot sit quietly in a classroom, read, or complete homework, they are not ready to return to competitive sports. Prioritizing return to learning for your child emphasizes the importance of academics but is also a real-world method of making sure that they have recovered from the concussion. Your child may be encouraged to gradually begin increasing physical activity under the supervision of a health care provider while they still have symptoms and need academic adjustment. They are not ready to return to competitive practice or games, however, if they still have symptoms in the classroom setting.

Academic Adjustments Following Concussion

Upon return to school, shorter days, reduced work demands, and other modifications will be important for the child or adolescent recovering from a concussion. Given the significant educational and social aspects of school, thoughtfully reintegrating your child or adolescent into the classroom is an important aspect of recovery. Although a limited number of students with more prolonged symptoms of concussion may require a formal education plan, such as an **Individualized Education Program (IEP)** or **504 plan** (Table 10.1), most students experiencing concussion symptoms benefit from informal academic adjustments and do not need a formal plan. Academic adjustments can be individually tailored to your child's symptoms and further adjusted as the child recovers. Examples of common general academic adjustments that may be recommended by the concussion recovery team include the following:

TABLE 10.1 504 Plans and Individualized Education Programs (IEPs)

Type of Plan	Description
504 plan	• Federally mandates academic accommodations to improve access to general education curriculum
IEP	• Part of the Individuals with Disabilities Education Act; ensures that students with disabilities receive an appropriate education • Considered a legal document that provides specialized interventions and special education for qualifying students

- Rest to manage symptoms
  - The student may initially need an excused absence from school for 1 or more days, depending on symptom severity.
  - Upon return to school, the student may need shorter days and for classes to be gradually added back into their schedule.
  - If the student feels worse in the morning, reintroduce afternoon classes first; if the student feels worse in the afternoon, reintroduce morning classes first.
  - Some students benefit from rest periods during the day. An ideal location is the school nurse's office or the athletic trainer's clinic. The school library can also provide respite from noise and stimulation and is a reasonable alternative if a nurse's office or clinic space is not available.
- Relaxed time demands
  - Deadlines for projects, papers, or other course assignments may need to be extended.
  - Multiple quizzes, tests, or examinations that are scheduled within a short time frame may need to be staggered or some tests delayed.

- o The student should be allowed extra time to complete in-class quizzes, tests, or examinations. "Time and a half" is a common modification and means that if a test is scheduled for 60 minutes, the student with concussion would have 90 minutes to complete it.
- o The student should be asked to complete a reduced number of test or homework items. For example, students recovering from concussion could be required to complete every other item instead of every item.
- Excused absence from physical education or alternate activities
  - o Participation in team-based activities or activities with significant physical exertion demands should not be allowed until the student has recovered and formal clearance has been obtained for return to play.
  - o The student should be allowed to rest quietly in the office of the nurse or guidance counselor, the library, or other quiet setting during physical education class.
  - o After the initial period of acute rest and once clearance to begin graded physical activity has been granted, allowing the student to walk during physical education class rather than participate in more strenuous activity is encouraged.
- Social activities
  - o As the student reintegrates into school and academic activity, they should also be encouraged to attend social events as tolerated. It may be best to delay participation in very loud and highly stimulating social activities during the early days after concussion.
  - o Students should be allowed visits from friends at home and not be isolated.
  - o Texting with friends and the use of social media is okay in moderation. Youth with visual symptoms may find extended use of smartphones uncomfortable and may self-limit the use of social technology.

o It is important not to isolate a child or adolescent with concussion symptoms. Allowing social contact with friends is an important aspect of normalcy and getting them back to their life.

Well-meaning health care providers have recommended extended periods of withdrawal and rest such that children and adolescents are confined to their rooms, absent from school, deprived of their smartphones and computers, and isolated from their friends. This "cocoon therapy" has resulted in prolonged recoveries because the children and adolescents become physically deconditioned because of lack of activity; they may also become depressed and anxious because of social isolation and extended absence from school. As a result, they start to worry and focus on their symptoms instead of getting better. As in adults, the goal is acute rest followed by gradual reintroduction into the typical and usual activities of daily living, including time with friends.

Academic Adjustments for Specific Concussion Symptoms

After concussion, some children and adolescents struggle with particularly problematic individual symptoms. As in adults, not all concussions in children and adolescents are the same, and some children or adolescents have greater difficulty with some symptoms and less or no difficulty with other symptoms. An individualized evaluation and tailored adjustments for academic activities can be very helpful in facilitating recovery. Be sure to discuss your child's symptoms with their health care provider or the management team that has been put in place to assist with your child's return to school. Some specific symptoms and academic adjustments may be recommended to help your child during recovery (Table 10.2).

TABLE 10.2 Specific Concussion Symptoms and Suggested Academic Adjustments

Symptom	How Symptom Affects Learning	Academic Adjustments
Headaches (the most common concussion symptom)	Can affect attention and concentration Pain levels may vary throughout the school day. Pain may be affected by school lighting (e.g., fluorescent lighting) and noise.	Allow frequent breaks for the student to close eyes or put head down on desk. Reduce overhead lighting or position the student to reduce the intensity of the light (e.g., sitting farther away from windows). Allow the student rest periods in the nurse's office or other quiet space. Allow excused absences from gym, band, choir, and assemblies and substitute rest periods or low-stimulation activities, such as sitting quietly in the library.
Dizziness/lightheadedness (may indicate vestibular dysfunction; check with your health care provider if this symptom is persisting to see if specialized treatment is needed)	Walking in crowded hallways or going up and down stairs may trigger symptoms. Symptoms may be triggered by visual stimulation, such as watching videos or computer screens.	Allow frequent breaks for the student to close eyes or put head down on desk. Allow the student to leave class early to get to their next class before hallways are crowded with other students.

TABLE 10.2 Continued

Symptom	How Symptom Affects Learning	Academic Adjustments
Visual symptoms (may include sensitivity to light, blurred vision, double vision, or eye strain/fatigue)	Eyes may fatigue easily with computer work or looking at smart boards. Symptoms may be triggered by visual stimulation, such as watching videos or computer screens.	Reduce overhead lighting or position the student to reduce the intensity of the light (i.e., sitting farther away from windows). Reduce the brightness level of electronic screens (e.g., laptops, tablets, smart boards) and use blue light filters on screens. Print a paper copy of computer-based materials for the student's review and study. Consider audio formats for the student instead of reading books.
Sound sensitivity	Loud noise may be uncomfortable. Excessive and prolonged auditory stimulation may make symptoms worse.	Allow the student to leave class early and get to their next class before hallways are crowded with other students. Allow the student to be excused from band, pep rallies, and other activities that increase symptoms.

Considerations for the College Student with Concussion

Although most college students are young adults rather than children or adolescents, some information is provided here as special considerations for "learners" after concussion. If you are a college student and think you may have a concussion, the university may have a student health clinic or infirmary where you can be evaluated. If the college or university does not have these resources, you may need to seek care from a health care provider in the community. If you are diagnosed with a concussion, you should request documentation from the school infirmary or clinic where you are evaluated so you can share it with your professors if needed. It is important to let your professors know about any specific academic recommendations you have been given by your health care provider. You should also contact your academic dean or your college's disability resource center and provide paperwork about any short-term academic adjustments your health care provider may have recommended to promote your recovery.

Fears About Falling Behind in School

While this information also applies to older students who are reading this book themselves, we will return to our focus in this chapter on providing information to parents who are helping their child navigate through a concussion. One important issue to be aware of is that your child or adolescent may become anxious about school and worried about their school performance after a concussion. Sometimes, the anxiety about their symptoms can make it feel as if their concussion symptoms are getting worse. Feeling flushed, sweaty, shaky, or lightheaded and experiencing heart racing or pounding are symptoms of anxiety that may feel just like concussion symptoms. For some youth, the anxiety can be more difficult to manage than the concussion itself. If you notice that your child seems anxious, worried, or stressed about school after a concussion, be positive and reassure them that they will feel much better soon and will be able to get back to their regular schoolwork and schedule. If your child does not seem reassured and the symptoms continue, talk to your child's health care provider or school psychologist. Working with a psychologist or neuropsychologist can help your child learn coping skills and strategies for managing anxiety.

Your Child's Return to Sports

If your child or adolescent is injured while playing a sport, they should be immediately removed from the sport and should not return to play until after they are evaluated by a health care professional who is knowledgeable about concussions. Your child should only return to sports participation after they have returned to learning and been cleared by a health care provider with expertise in concussion evaluation and management. Most states have specific guidelines for returning to sports for children enrolled in public high schools. In this case, your child's athletic trainer or other health care provider will need to provide the school with documentation stating that your child is medically cleared to begin the return-to-play process. However, policies may not be as well defined for younger children, for children participating in sports through non–school-based recreational leagues, or for children enrolled in private school. Parents may need to refer to the CDC guidelines and discuss the guidelines with health care providers to ensure that a return to play can occur as safely as possible.

Return to physical activity for children and adolescents after concussion is a gradual stepwise process in which light aerobic exercise is introduced first. If your child can participate in light aerobic exercise comfortably without worsening their concussion symptoms, more complex physical activities can be introduced. The next step involves adding in more complex physical activity of longer duration and intensity, such as playing pickup basketball or throwing a football with family members. If this increased activity is tolerated without increased symptoms, the next step is return to full physical activity. Keep in mind that although an adult with an uncomplicated recovery might be able to resume full physical activity in 1 week, some pediatric experts recommend that children take a couple of weeks or more to resume full physical activity, even those who are recovering well. Return to activity should always be an individual decision based on the specifics of your child's concussion, symptoms at time of injury, and clinical recovery.

It is common for parents to be worried about their child's return to playing sports after a concussion or about exposing their children to sports at all because of the increased risks of sustaining a concussion. It is important to remember, however, that well-managed concussions do not cause any lasting problems for the majority of individuals. In fact, a recent research study found that department chairs in neurosurgery and orthopedics had a higher rate of participating in contact sports in high school than other students. These high-achieving medical professionals also reported a high rate of having had at least one more concussion than the general population. In addition, participation in sports has multiple benefits for physical health, emotional well-being, and social development. In fact, from a population public health perspective, the health risks of obesity and inactivity are thought to be greater than the health risks of concussion. Encouraging physical activity and sports participation is important for healthy development. If you have worries about your child getting a concussion, talk with your child's health care provider and learn more about the safety plans and procedures for any sport you consider for your child. It is always important for parents to ask questions about all health and safety concerns related to their child's sports participation. It is also important to make sure your child's school or recreational league has a detailed concussion plan that includes education about concussion symptoms and to understand what resources are available if injury occurs, such as access to an athletic trainer or other health care re-sources. It is true that not all sports are created equal, and some sports are associated with a statistically greater number of concussions. Each family needs to make decisions about which sports and activities are best for their child as everyone has different abilities and comfort with different levels of risk. This is even true within families as some children may be more comfortable with higher-contact team sports while other children may prefer individual sports. More information about concussion and sports is provided in Chapter 12.

Summary

This chapter discussed how concussions are diagnosed and managed in children and provided information about the return-to-learn process. It is important to remember that your child's return to the classroom should be prioritized over their return to sport, with the expectation that they will return to all of their typical activities soon.

11

Can Having Attention-Deficit/Hyperactivity Disorder or a Learning Disorder Complicate Recovery from Concussion?

In this chapter, you will learn:

- The distinction between attention-deficit/hyperactivity disorder (ADHD) and learning disorders (sometimes called learning disabilities)
- Special considerations for those with ADHD and learning disorders who have a concussion

There has been debate among clinicians on whether having a **learning disorder** or a neurodevelopmental disorder such as **ADHD** may result in a prolonged recovery period from concussion. Let's start by defining the two terms and explaining how they are different. Both learning disorders (sometimes called **learning disabilities**) and ADHD are considered neurodevelopmental disorders, which means that they are evident from an early age and have a biological origin. Because both ADHD and learning disorders are often associated with school and school-aged children, many people assume they are just different types of learning disorders. Although both do affect learning, they are quite different. A learning disorder is when there are persisting difficulties with core academic skills, such as reading, writing, or math, that do not improve with standard academic supports. Clinicians and educators may use the term **specific learning disorder** to refer to a learning disability. Many people have heard the term **dyslexia**, which is an alternate term for a specific type of learning disorder affecting reading.

Children with learning disorders can focus their attention, but their brains have difficulty processing very specific types of important skills, such as reading. Although ADHD and learning disorders are present in childhood, the symptoms can persist into adulthood, and thus the information in this chapter is relevant to both children and adults.

In contrast to learning disorders, the key features of ADHD are predominant symptoms of inattention and/or hyperactivity and impulsivity. ADHD is associated with a variety of symptoms:

- Difficulty with attention and focus
- Problems with completing tasks and projects
- Struggles with organization
- Difficulty with sustained mental effort
- Losing or misplacing important items such as keys and smartphone
- Difficulty in keeping up with assignment deadlines and appointments
- Fidgeting and difficulty with staying seated or sitting quietly
- Restlessness or hyperactive behavior
- Talking excessively
- Blurting out answers in class or frequently interrupting others

It is important to understand that to be diagnosed with ADHD, these symptoms must have been present from an early age rather than beginning in adulthood or after an injury. If these symptoms occur after a traumatic brain injury, for example, they are symptoms of the brain injury and not of ADHD. The symptoms may be the same, but the cause is different.

Unfortunately, many research studies on concussion exclude people with a history of a learning disorder or other preexisting disorders, such as migraine headaches, to try to minimize factors other than concussion that could affect the results of the research study. As a result, our understanding of how some of these preexisting issues affect recovery outcome is not very well developed. Much of the research on concussion and learning disorders that has been done so far has focused on student-athletes with sports-related concussions. This research is often carried out using computerized cognitive tests, and many of these tests involve reading directions or rapidly processing symbols, which may be particularly difficult for someone with a learning disorder in reading or mathematics. Many of these research studies suggest that learning disorders affect student-athlete performance on computerized cognitive testing. Since these tests are used to track recovery from concussion, it is possible that it is not the learning disorder itself that delays recovery but that learning disorders affect performance on the measures used to track recovery.

Just as the symptoms of a learning disorder can make it difficult to track recovery from concussion using computerized cognitive tests, these clinical challenges also occur with ADHD. As discussed earlier in this chapter, common symptoms of ADHD include difficulty with attention, concentration, and focus, as well as impulsivity and hyperactivity. Individuals with ADHD may also have a hard time regulating their behaviors or emotions, being timely, completing tasks, or staying organized. Any or all of these symptoms of ADHD may result in errors or other difficulties on computerized cognitive testing, and it can be difficult to sort out these preexisting symptoms of ADHD that may look just like concussion symptoms on these tests. Because some of these symptoms and core features of ADHD—especially sustained attention and difficulty concentrating—are similar to symptoms of concussion, it is important to discuss your history of ADHD and use of medications for ADHD with your clinician.

Because ADHD or a learning disorder can affect performance on commonly used computerized tests used to track concussion recovery, it is important to be evaluated by a clinician, such as a neuropsychologist, with expertise in untangling these factors. Everyone's recovery after concussion is individual, and not everyone with ADHD or a learning disorder will experience a longer recovery period or have difficulty on this computerized testing. More research is needed to understand how—or if—having ADHD or a learning disorder might affect your recovery if you have a concussion.

Griffin is a high school student who plays on a lacrosse team. He was always very active as a child and often got into trouble at school for blurting out answers without being called on by the teacher and for leaving his seat and running around in the classroom. He was diagnosed with ADHD when he was in elementary school and started taking medication, which helped him concentrate better at school and stay focused while completing tasks at home. His energy has served him well on the sports field, and he is a tremendous athlete. He is one of the best players on his lacrosse team, and he really enjoys competing, although sometimes his competitiveness gets him into trouble.

One day during practice, his teammate starts trash-talking after breezing past him and several other defenders to score a goal. Griffin has a hard time controlling his reactions in situations like this, and he escalates things with his teammate until his teammate eventually tackles him, knocking him to the ground with a lot of force. The athletic trainer sees what has happened and goes over to make sure that Griffin is okay. Griffin has a hard time getting up off the ground because he feels woozy and as if he is going to get sick. He ends up vomiting several times. After a brief assessment, the athletic trainer decides that it is best for Griffin to be evaluated in the emergency department.

In the emergency department, he is taken for a CT scan of the brain, which does not show any abnormalities. He is diagnosed with a concussion and told to go home and rest. He is also told to stop taking his ADHD medication until he can be cleared by a neurologist. He can't get in to see the neurologist for about a week and a half, and in the meantime, he is having a really hard time in most of his classes. He forgets to turn in assignments and finds it almost impossible to concentrate during the lectures for his online class. He feels more scattered than he has felt in a long time and is starting to get really down on himself and worried that this concussion will set him back.

When he sees the neurologist, he learns that it is safe for him to start taking his ADHD medication again and that he likely never needed to stop taking it in the first place. Griffin starts to feel a lot more like himself again after he restarts his medication, and he is able to start the return-to-play process under the supervision of his athletic trainer.

ADHD may be a risk factor for concussion, meaning that individuals with ADHD are more likely than others to sustain a concussion, because they are more likely to be impulsive and take risks. In fact, people with ADHD may be more likely to have injuries of all kinds. While it does not appear that having ADHD prolongs the recovery process after concussion, it can present some additional challenges at school or work, though, during the period of recovery.

Concussion may temporarily make it more difficult for those with ADHD or other neurodevelopmental disorders to use their existing organizational strategies to help them stay on task toward achieving a goal. These strategies include setting timers or calendar alerts, making lists of steps to follow, or color-coding school or work materials. When you are not feeling like yourself, it can be more difficult to do things that require more effort or are naturally harder for you. This is particularly true if you have ADHD. It may be much harder to use your organizational and **self-monitoring** skills after a concussion, so it might feel even more difficult to manage your concussion than it might be for someone without ADHD.

A concussion can temporarily worsen the symptoms of ADHD or amplify the challenges associated with a learning disorder. As a result, students may need additional academic adjustments or modifications to their academic plan, such as an Individualized Education Program (IEP) or 504 plan, during their recovery. These academic plans and suggested academic adjustments are described in detail in Chapter 10. Adults with ADHD or a learning disorder may find that they need to allow additional time to complete work tasks and require additional structure in their work while they are recovering.

Many people with ADHD take stimulant medication to help them focus and improve their other symptoms. If you take medication for ADHD, it is very important to keep taking your ADHD medication consistently after concussion so that any concussion-related changes in cognitive functioning can be identified and tracked over time. If you stop taking your ADHD medication after a concussion, it can be difficult to monitor your cognitive recovery and understand whether the cognitive changes you are experiencing are a result of the concussion or an increase in your ADHD symptoms. In addition, ADHD symptoms can result in increased risk-taking behaviors or lapses in attention or focus, making secondary concussions more likely, so staying on prescribed ADHD medication following a concussion can be vital in preventing additional injury because of inattention or risk-taking.

Summary

ADHD and learning disorders are both neurodevelopmental disorders that can affect academic performance and many other aspects of life. For adults with ADHD or learning disorders, the symptoms can affect work performance and social relationships. Whereas learning disorders affect processing of very specific skills, such as reading or math, ADHD symptoms include difficulty with attention and/or hyperactivity and impulsivity. Research suggests that

ADHD and learning disorders are associated with a longer recovery period after concussion, but it appears that this finding may be related to how these disorders affect performance on the tools used to track recovery. Because research studies on concussion often exclude participants with learning disorders and ADHD, much remains to be learned.

12

Athletes and Sport-Related Concussions

In this chapter, you will learn:

- Why special procedures for sport-related concussions are important
- How sport-related concussions are evaluated and managed
- Why helmets and safety equipment are important
- Why avoiding multiple concussions is critical
- When to consider retiring from sport

Why have a special chapter on concussion in athletes? Many sports have increased risk of concussion because the nature of the sport involves collisions or fast-paced action that might result in injuries, including concussions. An important goal is to maximize the health benefits of sports and recreational activities and reduce the risks, including the risk of concussion. It is extremely important that anyone participating in contact sports or sports with a risk of injury (which is just about all of them) be completely recovered from concussion before resuming contact play or competition. Getting a second concussion before recovering from the first concussion can cause significantly worse symptoms and a longer recovery period. Because of these concerns, special safety procedures have been established for managing concussions in athletes. This chapter discusses how sport-related concussions are evaluated and managed at various levels of sports participation and examines some important considerations for the athlete who has sustained more than one concussion through participation in sports.

Kira is a high school sophomore and a competitive swimmer at the state level. She is in the pool for warmup at a high school swim meet when she takes an elbow to the side of her head from the swimmer in the next lane over. She feels woozy and sick to her stomach immediately. Her swim coach sees what happens and whistles for everyone to stop swimming so that Kira can safely get out of the pool to be evaluated by the on-staff athletic trainer. Kira is embarrassed that everyone has to stop swimming and insists that she is fine. The athletic trainer walks with her to a quiet area where she is evaluated. She tells the athletic trainer that she feels okay, although she is feeling nauseated and somewhat off balance. She is really hoping to be able to compete that evening, especially because it is one of her last chances to qualify for the state championship meet. The athletic trainer proceeds to evaluate her, assessing her awareness, thinking skills, and balance. Kira is informed that she has likely sustained a concussion and that she will not be able to participate in the remainder of the swim meet.

There has been a great deal of positive attention and progress made in increasing awareness of concussion safety in sports, resulting in new protocols and policies to protect athletes' health. Because many of us enjoy watching sports and seeing the impressive physical accomplishments of professional or elite amateur athletes, we tend to follow news stories about athletes closely. Athletes who have sustained concussions have had a great deal of media exposure and it is natural to feel empathy and concern for them. Due to the media coverage, some athletes or parents of athletes may be left wondering if participation in sports is safe. Some sports do have an inherently increased concussion risk because of their high levels of athlete-to-athlete contact. These sports are called contact sports and include American football, ice hockey, and rugby. However, concussions can also occur in sports in which less contact typically occurs, such as in swimming. For this reason, it is important that all athletes (even those participating in noncontact sports) learn about the signs and symptoms of concussion and understand what the return-to-sport-participation process may look like.

Although some critics have called for ending specific sports because of concerns about increased concussion risk, it is important to realize the significant physical, emotional, and social benefits of playing organized sports. Also, careful research by scientists on how concussions occur in sport has resulted in rule changes that have been implemented in contact sports such as American football and ice hockey to reduce the risk of injury. In addition, the heightened awareness of concussion safety at all levels of sport has resulted in legislation that promotes safe participation in athletics. Every U.S. state and the District of Columbia now has some form of concussion legislation for youth (public high school) athletes that requires removal from activity to evaluate for concussion. Immediately removing a youth athlete from sport in the event of a suspected concussion—and prohibiting return to that sport on the same day as the injury—is a cornerstone of most legislation. Professional, college, and even some high school sports also have concussion protocols to improve player safety. Although differences exist in the number of resources available for implementing concussion protocols across various levels of sports, from youth sports to collegiate sports and professional leagues, the protocols have some common features.

Evaluating Concussions in the Sport Setting

A variety of health care providers who are unique to the sport setting may be involved in diagnosing and managing sport-related concussions. Because some of these professionals are likely to be involved in the initial diagnosis, it's important to understand their roles. It is also important to note that sports teams differ in their access to the types of health care providers who specialize in the evaluation and management of sports concussion. If you or your child participates in sports, it may be helpful to identify who these health care providers are and ask them about their process of evaluating and managing sport-related concussions.

At the high school level, access to care varies widely depending on the financial resources available across different school districts. Many athletes are evaluated by a **certified athletic trainer** (**athletic trainer** for short), a skilled professional who has extensive training in working with other health care professionals to identify and manage injuries that occur in sports. In addition to extensive training in on-the-field or on-the-court diagnosis of a variety of sports-related orthopedic injuries, athletic trainers also have specialized education and training in recognizing, diagnosing, and managing sport-related concussions. High school sports teams may have athletic trainers at practices and games or may have a centralized location where the athletic trainer is located in the event an injury occurs. Other schools may evaluate and manage concussions through volunteer physicians, coaches, school nurses, or other trained personnel.

When a concussion is diagnosed by a certified athletic trainer or other trained professional, the athlete is referred to a licensed health care provider for further evaluation and written clearance for return to the activity. At the middle school or high school level, the provider may be a pediatrician or family doctor who has experience with concussion. At the collegiate level, a **sports medicine physician** may provide the evaluation. In many school systems and various levels of sports, a neuropsychologist or **sports neuropsychologist** evaluates and manages athletes with sport-related concussion injuries. The athlete may also be seen by a **sports neurologist**, a neurologist with subspecialty training related to sport-related neurologic injuries. Each of these health care providers has different areas of clinical expertise, but all play a valuable role in keeping athletes safe in the context of an injury. Further information about these professionals is provided in Table 12.1.

Athletic trainers are typically on the sidelines during sports practices and events and may be the first individuals to notice an

TABLE 12.1 Health Care Providers with Specialized Training in Management of Sport-Related Injuries

Provider Type	Training and Expertise
Athletic trainer	Extensive training in on-the-field or on-the-court diagnosis of a variety of sport-related injuries, including concussion. Athletic trainers typically have a bachelor's or master's degree and work under the supervision of a physician. About 70% have a master's degree, and some have a doctorate.
Sports neurologist	Physicians with expertise in brain-based and nervous system medical disorders and specialized training in sport-related neurologic injuries. Sports neurologists have a medical degree and specialty residency training in neurologic disorders followed by fellowship training in sports neurology.
Sports neuropsychologist	Clinical neuropsychologists with experience in applying knowledge of brain–behavior relationships to the evaluation and treatment of sports-related brain injury. Sports neuropsychologists complete a doctorate degree followed by specialized fellowship training in neuropsychology.
Sports medicine physician	Physicians with specialty training in musculoskeletal injuries and common medical conditions that affect those with a physically active lifestyle and athletic participation. Sports medicine physicians have a medical degree and specialty residency training in family medicine, orthopedics, or physical medicine and rehabilitation followed by a fellowship in sports medicine.

athlete is showing signs of concussion. The athletic trainer or other trained medical professional first checks for signs of very serious injury that may require emergency medical services and transport to the nearest hospital emergency department. Fortunately, in most situations, the athlete is able to walk off the field or court and undergoes further evaluation on the sidelines or pool deck, in the locker room, or in another area away from the game action.

During a sideline evaluation for concussion, the athlete will be evaluated for symptoms of concussion and observed again for signs of more severe injury. If any red flags are seen that indicate a deteriorating condition, such as decreased alertness, seizure, a headache increasing in severity (especially if associated with vomiting), and/or double vision, a thorough evaluation is critical to determine whether transport to a hospital emergency department is needed. The athletic trainer or other trained medical professional will conduct an evaluation using a standardized protocol. One commonly used structured evaluation is called the **Sport Concussion Assessment Tool—5th Edition (SCAT5)**. The SCAT5 provides a formal procedure for evaluating current symptoms of concussion, including symptoms reported by the athlete, such as headaches, dizziness, blurred vision, and balance problems. As part of this evaluation, the athlete will then be formally evaluated with a brief cognitive screening that typically includes the following:

- A short series of orientation questions to determine whether the athlete knows basic information such as the time, day, date, and year
- Evaluation of attention and concentration skills by having the athlete repeat back increasing strings of numbers backwards
- Testing of immediate memory by asking the athlete to listen to and repeat a series of words three times
- A brief neurologic evaluation and balance assessment, followed by asking the athlete to repeat the list of words learned earlier

The SCAT5 has a scoring and decision component to aid in the diagnosis of concussion; however, it cannot be overemphasized that the SCAT5 and other concussion evaluation tools are simply that—tools used as diagnostic aids. This means that the person evaluating the athlete will use this or other tools combined with their clinical expertise to make a diagnosis. The certified athletic trainer or other professional will also consider any preexisting medical conditions or other preinjury factors that may play a role in how the athlete performs on sideline testing, such as a history of learning disabilities or preexisting headache syndromes. Remember, concussion is a clinical diagnosis and not just a label based on a checklist or assessment tool. It is also important to know that the SCAT is revised and updated on a regular basis based on current best clinical practices and scientific evidence so in the future you may see a SCAT6 or other name for this or similar measures.

If the clinician performing the sideline evaluation determines that a concussion has occurred, the athlete will be removed from play and not returned to practice or competition for the remainder of the day to allow for more thorough evaluation. If a concussion is suspected, immediate removal from play is critically important to minimize the risk of more severe and catastrophic injury. The most devastating outcomes in sport concussion injuries occur when an athlete sustains a concussion, even a mild concussive injury, and then returns to the same game and sustains another hit (or hits) while the brain is still vulnerable from the initial injury. Although the exact mechanism is unclear, the outcome can be devastating because of brain swelling inside the skull (with or without bleeding in the brain), compressing the part of the brain that regulates vital life functions and resulting in death or severe neurologic injury. This rare devastating reaction from subsequent injuries before recovery is known as **second impact syndrome**.

The true story of Zackery Lystedt highlights the importance of being evaluated and removed from game play after a suspected concussion. Zackery Lystedt was a 13-year-old football player who experienced a devastating neurologic injury when he returned to a game after an earlier hit that produced concussion symptoms. He collapsed on the field and was airlifted to a nearby medical center, where he underwent neurosurgical procedures to relieve rapid swelling of his brain and had several **strokes**. Zackery required prolonged hospitalization and rehabilitation, was in a coma for 3 months, and was unable to speak a word for 9 months. This talented multisport athlete was not able to stand without assistance for nearly 3 years after his injury. Zackery and his parents are remarkable for the strength they exhibited throughout Zackery's recovery and for their advocating for the protection of other youth athletes through enactment of concussion safety legislation. In 2009, the Zackery Lystedt Law was passed in Washington State; it was the first comprehensive youth sports concussion legislation and the model for legislation in other states. Fortunately, such devastating injuries are very rare, but they highlight the importance of evaluating any athlete even suspected of having a concussion and preventing that athlete from returning to play the same day.

Reporting Suspected Concussions

Many sports programs now educate their athletes about concussion symptoms during the preseason each year, reviewing what the symptoms are and the importance of telling the athletic trainer if they think they may have sustained a concussion so a proper evaluation can be performed. Athletes are usually made aware that research has shown that failing to immediately report a suspected concussion can result in a longer recovery period and more time out of their sport. Despite this, some athletes still do not report suspected concussions for a number of reasons. Many athletes may mistake their concussion symptoms for other familiar issues, such as dehydration or fatigue. Others may hesitate to tell anyone about their suspected concussion out of fear of judgment or reduced playing time. Some athletes may also perceive pressure from their teammates or coaches to continue playing, even if they are hurt. This is why medical professionals who diagnose and manage concussion often rely on tools such as cognitive and balance assessments for making decisions about concussion and return to play rather than exclusively relying on an athlete's reported symptoms.

If you are an athlete and think you may have just gotten a concussion, it is important to inform the coach and athletic trainer immediately and to be absolutely honest about any symptoms you may be experiencing. It is normal to feel worried about getting playing time, the outcome of the game or event, or what the coach may think, but it is always more important to prioritize health above all else. It is also important to tell the athletic trainer or other medical professionals if you feel extra pressure from coaches to return to play. It is the responsibility of the coaching staff to work together with the athletic trainer and other members of the medical team to get athletes back to playing as quickly and safely as possible.

The Role of Baseline Evaluations

If you are participating in sports, you may have had to undergo a concussion baseline evaluation. Baseline evaluations are assessments of concussion-related symptoms conducted before a concussion has occurred and typically before sports participation has started for the season. Preseason baseline evaluations can make it easier for health care professionals to identify a concussion when it occurs because they have information about what the athlete was like before the concussion. This information can help them detect subtle changes in thinking, balance, and other symptoms. Baseline evaluations may look different depending on the type of sport and level of participation (youth, collegiate, professional). Baseline evaluations are most commonly carried out in contact sports or sports in which concussions are most common, but they may also be recommended for all athletes at some levels of training (such as collegiate) and may be required as part of a yearly physical examination before the start of the sport season.

If you are an athlete participating in a baseline concussion evaluation, you will likely be asked about any symptoms you normally have or have at the time of the evaluation. For example, you may be asked if you have headaches and how often. You will also likely participate in a brief assessment of your thinking skills. These assessments are often done on a computer and can be completed relatively quickly, usually within around 25 minutes. You may also participate in a balance assessment to see how well you can balance while holding different poses and on different surfaces. Depending on the school or athletic system, other assessments may also be incorporated into the baseline evaluations, including more comprehensive and sophisticated balance assessment, visual tracking, or questionnaires that ask about a variety of physical and emotional symptoms.

If you or your child are participating in sports, you may want to ask the certified athletic trainer or coaching staff about baseline concussion assessment. Baseline assessment can be particularly important when the athlete experiences headaches, balance problems, or other concussion-type symptoms at baseline (before injury). If there is a history of learning problems, a neurodevelopmental disorder such as attention-deficit/hyperactivity disorder (ADHD), or a preexisting medical or psychological condition that overlaps with concussion symptoms, it is particularly important to ask about baseline evaluations. At a minimum, always make sure that the certified athletic trainer or team sports medicine physician is aware of any of preexisting medical condition you may have so they can take it into account when assessing for a suspected concussion and monitoring your recovery.

Return to Sport

It is important to understand that returning to your sport is very different from returning to general physical activity. Although beginning to resume physical activity such as walking 2 to 3 days after a concussion is encouraged for everyone, including athletes, it is critically important that a special protocol described below is followed before returning to athletic competition or full participation in sports to reduce the likelihood of more severe brain injury. After a concussion, athletes will not be able to return to sport until they have fully recovered from the injury and have been evaluated and cleared by a licensed health care provider with experience in concussion evaluation and management. Research has shown that trying to rush back into sports participation can actually complicate and prolong the recovery process, and athletes should never return to playing sports the same day that they have been diagnosed with a concussion, as demonstrated in Zackery Lystedt's story.

How do you know when it is safe to return to play? The most widely used protocol to guide decisions about return to sport was developed by the Concussion in Sport Group (CISG). The CISG is an international group of experts who typically meet every few years to review and update recommendations and guidelines for the management of sport concussion. Based on a thorough review of the most current research, the guidelines are updated at each meeting to incorporate evidence-based approaches to the management of athletes with concussion. For example, the meeting held in Berlin, Germany, in 2016 resulted in recommendations that are often called the Berlin Guidelines, and these have been adopted by many other countries and organizations. These guidelines outline a stepwise approach to gradually resuming physical activity and participation in sports after an initial 24- to 48-hour period of rest. If you are an athlete with a concussion, your health care providers and certified athletic trainer or other trained professionals will work through this stepwise approach with you while carefully monitoring your symptoms. The steps are important for all athletes, family members, and friends to keep in mind when a concussion has been diagnosed. The recommended steps for return to play outlined in widely used guidelines are:

1. Gradually reintroducing daily activities that do not worsen symptoms

2. Starting light aerobic activity such as walking or stationary cycling
3. Adding sport-specific running or skating drills
4. Introducing more complex training drills, including progressive resistance training
5. Allowing return to normal contact practice after medical clearance
6. Returning to competition/game participation

Current guidelines are designed to safely reintroduce monitored activity and return to sport. Each step listed in the return-to-play process is recommended to take at least 24 hours for adult athletes. If your symptoms increase or recur with additional physical exertion, you should go back to the previous stage of activity. Once you have progressed through the first four steps without a recurrence of the concussion symptoms, you can be medically cleared to resume practice and then competition. As part of a clearance to return to play, the health care team may want to repeat the computer-based cognitive testing and balance assessment you took at baseline to ensure you are performing at the same level as on the preseason testing.

According to the 2016 international concussion guidelines, an athlete with a fairly uneventful recovery will typically require at least 7 days until they are cleared for return to competition. If symptoms last longer than 10 to 14 days, further evaluation by a health care provider with expertise in sports concussion is recommended. As clinical research accumulates, the length of time required for recovery before return to sport may increase and there may be new recommendations from the next CISG meeting. It should be noted that youth athletes may need a longer period of time between each step of the progression (see Chapter 10). Some pediatric neurologists recommend that younger athletes take a minimum of 48 hours between each step, whereas adult athletes may only need 24 hours between steps. Youth or adult athletes with a history of previous concussions or preexisting medical conditions such as migraine headaches may also need a longer period of recovery between steps.

For student athletes, an important consideration in Return-to-Sport decisions is whether the student athlete has first been able to resume their academic studies to the same level as prior to the injury. A full discussion of Return to Learning considerations is in Chapter 10.

Helmets and Safety Equipment

Proper use of helmets and safety equipment is essential in minimizing injury. It is important to realize, however, that helmets do not eliminate the risk of concussion. Helmets were designed to protect against skull fracture and more severe head injury. To reduce sport-specific injuries, it is critically important to use safety equipment and follow the safety rules required by each sport. It is also important that the helmets be properly fitted, well maintained, age appropriate, and certified for use in that sport and position. Many different helmet types are available, even within the same sport. For example, baseball batters and catchers wear different helmets, and hockey goalies wear helmets that are distinct from the rest of their team. Helmets that are cracked, broken, or altered in any way should never be used, and chin straps should be properly fitted and used. Box 12.1 provides a summary of helmet care. For additional safety information and sport-specific helmet information, refer to the U.S. Centers for Disease Control and Prevention fact sheets (available at https://www.cdc.gov/headsup/helmets/index.html).

Some athletes or their parents have inquired about using helmets or other forms of headgear while participating in sports in which helmets are not customarily worn. Although some products on the market are geared toward "reducing concussion risk," the research on the efficacy of these products is mixed. In sports in which helmets

---

BOX 12.1 **Helmet Care and Safety**

- Always check the exterior and interior of the helmet for any signs of cracks, broken pieces, or damaged padding.
- Do not use damaged helmets.
- Do not throw, sit, or stand on the helmet.
- Do not store the helmet in a hot car. Store it away from direct sunlight.
- Keep the helmet clean with gentle detergent and hand cleansing.
- Do not affix stickers or other unapproved items to the helmet. These might affect the integrity of the helmet and violate the manufacturer's warranty.

---

are not worn by athletes, such as field hockey or soccer, any extra protective gear worn must be in compliance with league or sport regulations and must always be used under the direct supervision of the certified athletic trainer and/or other health care providers.

Multiple Concussions

Some youth, amateur, and professional athletes sustain multiple concussions during their athletic careers. If properly managed using the accepted concussion management guidelines, most athletes have no long-lasting effects from multiple concussions. The most important factor for a positive outcome is to make sure that the athlete recovered fully before returning to contact practice and competition. Research indicates that the period of greatest vulnerability for sustaining a second concussion is in the first 10 days after a concussion, so making sure an athlete has returned to baseline and achieved clinical recovery is key. If an athlete sustains concussions that are well spread out, with full recovery between each concussion, the long-term risk appears to be small. When an athlete sustains a concussion while they are still recovering from a previous concussion, however, the risk of more serious injury and the cumulative effects of multiple concussions increase. For this reason, it is absolutely critical that athletes be honest with health care providers about any prior concussions. If you have questions about the relationship between multiple concussions and chronic traumatic encephalopathy (CTE), please refer back to Chapter 9.

Retirement from Sport

Determining when to retire an athlete from sport is a difficult, complex, and important decision. Sports are an important part of life for many of us, and for many athletes, their identity—and sometimes financial stability—is rooted in their sports participation. Nevertheless, several indicators suggest strong consideration of retirement from sport:

- Persisting neurologic symptoms, such as changes in thinking, headaches, or balance, that do not return to the athlete's baseline level of functioning
- Cognitive weaknesses on neuropsychological testing that suggest persisting symptoms that are not resolving
- Progressively longer periods required for recovery after each subsequent concussion
- Exposure to less force resulting in concussion symptoms of greater intensity
- Neuroimaging evidence of structural damage

Retirement decisions should never be taken lightly and should always involve consideration of the potential positives and negatives associated with prolonged sports participation. Interdisciplinary evaluation, consultation, and care is recommended in such situations to ensure a thorough and thoughtful evaluation and discussion of risks with the athlete. Sports neuropsychologists are an important part of this interdisciplinary team. In addition to evaluating the cumulative effect of concussions on thinking abilities, sports neuropsychologists can support athletes as they navigate retirement from sport and explore other identities and roles. Sports psychologists or other mental health providers may also assist the athlete with this difficult transition.

Summary

This chapter discussed how concussions that occur in the context of sports are evaluated, the internationally recognized guidelines for returning to sport after a concussion, the unique pressures athletes may face after a suspected concussion, and the importance of reporting suspected concussions to athletic trainers, coaches, or other professionals. Many athletes experience one or more sports concussions in their lifetime; if properly managed, these cause no long-lasting effects for most athletes. Proper use of safety equipment and following safety rules can reduce the likelihood of concussion. Any athlete concerned about the cumulative effects of concussions or exposure to subconcussive forces should seek a comprehensive neurologic and neuropsychological evaluation. Evidence of an increasingly prolonged recovery period, or increased symptoms with progressively less impact force, may signal the need for retirement from sport.

13

Occupational and Work Issues Related
to Concussion

In this chapter, you will learn:

- How to navigate going back to work following a concussion
- How going back to work can impact aspects of recovery
- How to discuss your concussion with your employer
- What workers' compensation is and how it works

As discussed in Chapter 1, it is important to promptly seek medical attention after a suspected concussion. If you are an employee, this is particularly important so that you can get the support you need as you navigate the process of returning to work after an injury. It is important to inform your health care team about the type of work you do and what your schedule is so specific recommendations about return to work can be provided as part of your evaluation. Prompt evaluation is also important so you can receive any necessary treatment and get back to work as quickly and safely as possible. Chapters 3, 4, and 5 discussed the early symptoms of concussion and how specific symptoms can be managed to promote recovery. Depending on the nature of your work, it may be helpful or necessary to take some time off. This will depend on the symptoms you experience early in your recovery and the extent to which your symptoms increase at work or make it difficult to complete job-related tasks. The safety of yourself and others is an important consideration. For example, if you operate heavy machinery, you should not return to that specific work task until you have fully recovered and been cleared by a health care provider.

Once your early symptoms have decreased, however, or are being appropriately managed and monitored by your health care team, efforts should be made for you to gradually return to work as soon as possible. Initially, this might mean working for short intervals at a time (e.g., 15 to 30 minutes) followed by rest breaks, and then gradually increasing to longer periods of part-time work as tolerated until you are able to work a full day. If your work involves potentially dangerous activities, such as operating heavy machinery or working with high-voltage power lines, you may be able to return to doing some parts of your job; however, as noted above, you should not engage in dangerous activities until you have been cleared by an experienced health care provider. Extended periods of time out of work can result in cognitive deconditioning (see Chapter 8), as well as physical deconditioning. In addition, if you stay out of work for a long period of time, you will likely have new financial stress because of the lack of income and possibly stress in your relationships. All this additional stress, along with the social isolation and cognitive and physical deconditioning that come with being out of work, can make it feel as if your concussion symptoms are worsening. Concussion symptoms can be very similar to the symptoms of stress, and extra stress can negatively impact your recovery process.

Natalia is a 42-year-old mother of two who works full time as a retail sales associate. On the weekends, she also helps take care of her father, who is ill, and her aunt, who has late-stage dementia. Natalia is finishing up at work one morning after an overnight shift to help with a large shipment. She is placing merchandise when she accidentally bangs her head hard against a metal display shelf. Immediately after hitting her head, Natalia feels dazed. On top of the exhaustion she is already feeling, she now feels dizzy, off balance, and as if she is in a fog. With just a few minutes left in her shift, Natalia leaves work. Over the next 2 days, Natalia experiences ongoing symptoms that prompt her

> *to make an appointment with her primary care doctor. Her doctor conducts a thorough evaluation and gives her some exercises to help with her balance problems and dizziness. Natalia's doctor insists that it is not safe for her to return to work, where she often climbs ladders to reach displays, until her symptoms are better controlled. Natalia's doctor provides her with relevant paperwork and encourages her to contact her employer to discuss her options for taking some time off.*

Although returning to work as soon as possible after a concussion is generally a good idea, returning to work after a concussion is not without unique challenges and complexities. Most of the acute symptoms of concussion, whether cognitive, emotional, or physical in nature, have the potential to negatively affect your work performance. For example, if you are experiencing concentration difficulties and slowed thinking, you may have a difficult time in a fast-paced work setting that requires rapid decision-making and high levels of productivity. The compensatory strategies listed in Chapter 8 may be helpful for your return to work; you may need additional time to complete your work, a written list of your "to-do" items at work each day, or written instructions for any new job tasks. If you experience anxiety or increased irritability in the context of a concussion, you may have difficulty in a work setting that requires frequent interpersonal communication and problem solving, such as a job in human resources, social work, or health care. If your concussion resulted in fatigue, balance problems, or visual disturbance, physically demanding jobs such as retail stock work, construction, or nursing may be more difficult or even unsafe for you and those around you.

Given that work settings may worsen the symptoms of concussion and that your symptoms may negatively affect your productivity at work, it is very important to maintain an open dialogue with your employer to discuss available options. It is important to realize that although federal and state legislature is in place to protect your rights as an employee, not all employers are created equal in terms of their specific policies. Despite increased societal attention, concussion is often misunderstood by employers. Your employer may not understand the injury itself, the way it can affect your work performance, or your need to take time away from work. Ask your health care team for documentation to describe your current symptoms and any potential risks associated with returning to work. This documentation may also include a return-to-work plan that outlines any special adjustments or work modifications to help you smoothly transition back into your typical work routine. You should also arrange a meeting with your supervisor and human resources (HR) personnel to discuss the plan, provide and receive appropriate paperwork, and gauge your employer's willingness to support you during this transitional period. If you are nervous about speaking with your employer or supervisor, it can be helpful to role-play the conversation with a friend or to make a list of talking points to bring with you along with any paperwork from your medical team.

Josh is a 22-year-old research assistant in a neuroscience laboratory who sustains a concussion while playing Ultimate Frisbee with friends one Friday after work. Josh really enjoys his work and is highly motivated to perform well since he is applying to medical school and needs a strong letter of recommendation. However, after his injury, Josh is feeling really groggy and has a hard time focusing. He also finds it difficult to get a good night's sleep and is struggling with headaches. After 2 nights without sleep, Josh experiences a flurry of anxiety about going back to work on Monday. He isn't sure how he will carry out his typical work tasks and fears that his supervisor will think differently of him if he isn't able to "push through." Eventually he sends an email to his supervisor explaining what happened and requesting a time to meet with her. He writes down the things that he wants to say in the meeting so that he can refer to his talking points if he gets distracted or nervous in the moment. His supervisor ends up being extremely supportive and works with him to identify tasks he feels confident doing while he is still recovering. She encourages him to take breaks throughout the day as needed and follow any specific recommendations from his health care team. The following day, Josh is seen at a concussion clinic, where he is given a lot of reassurance that he is recovering well from his injury. He is provided with a formal plan for returning to his typical work activities based on observations and testing that is carried out as part of the appointment. He discusses this plan with his supervisor, who remains supportive during his recovery process. By the following week, Josh is back to his typical work activities and is feeling totally back to normal.

When you are ready to talk with your employer about your concussion, these tips can be very helpful:

- Request a private meeting with your supervisor or employer to talk about your injury.
- Ask your supervisor if HR should be included in this first meeting.
- Ask your health care provider to give you a letter for your employer that briefly describes your injury and symptoms that might affect your ability to work.
- If your employer requires special forms to be completed by your health care provider, be sure the forms are completed and bring them to the meeting.
- Talk with your supervisor about any aspects of your job that might need to be modified during your return to work.
- Ask your supervisor how best to coordinate any modifications you need with HR. Your supervisor may recommend you coordinate with HR for all future discussions about your recovery. Each employer is different, so it is important to ask the procedure you should follow for your company or organization.

One of the challenges you may encounter is that, depending on your employer's specific policies and or preferences, it might be difficult to arrange a gradual return-to-work plan. Some employers have an all-or-nothing approach when it comes to supporting an injured employee. These employers may be less willing to provide special support or accommodations and may not feel comfortable with you returning to work if you are not able to maintain your preinjury level of work performance. The employer may insist that you use sick leave or vacation time for any days missed or may require that you file for formal medical leave, during which you may or may not be paid. In the United States, the **Family and Medical Leave Act (FMLA)** is in place to protect an injured employee's job for up to 12 weeks per year, meaning that the injured employee cannot be terminated or replaced during that time frame. Medical leave through FMLA is unpaid, although the employee's health benefits are maintained throughout the leave period. General qualifications for FMLA eligibility are listed on the U.S. Department of Labor website (*dol.gov/agencies/whd/fmla*) and include the following:

- You must have worked for your employer for at least 12 months.
- You must have worked at least 1250 hours over the past 12 months.
- You must work for an employer that employs at least 50 people within a 75-mile radius.

If your symptoms are prolonged or particularly debilitating, your doctor or health care team may refer you to work with a **vocational rehabilitation specialist**. Vocational rehabilitation specialists are able to determine the specific physical, cognitive, and emotional requirements of a particular job and can assess the extent to which you can currently meet those demands. Vocational rehabilitation specialists or occupational therapists can work with you to facilitate a smooth transition back to work. Vocational rehabilitation assessments typically involve directly observing you during an office visit or in your home or workplace to gather meaningful information about your current abilities, work duties, work-related interests, and ability to participate in leisure activities. Findings from the assessment are used to shape interventions that will help you get back to work. If you are no longer able to participate in your profession, vocational rehabilitation specialists can also help you identify alternative employment possibilities.

If you sustain a concussion at work, some additional options may be available. In most states, employees who are injured at work or while carrying out work-related duties may be able to make a claim for participation in a compensation system called **workers' compensation**. This system helps protect injured employees from some of the negative financial consequences of an injury. Injured employees who are unable to work because of their symptoms may be entitled to receive up to two-thirds of any lost wages during their leave period. In addition, injured employees may have their medical and rehabilitation care paid for by their employer or their medical insurance. If you were injured on the job doing work-related activities, your employer may refer you to an occupational medicine provider to help document and treat your work-related injuries.

An important aspect of workers' compensation to be aware of involves the protection of privacy of medical records provided by a law known as the Health Care Portability and Accountability Act (**HIPAA**). Ordinarily, this law protects your rights to privacy as you seek medical care, and it means that your personal medical records have special protection. However, if you apply for workers' compensation, several agencies or groups may be involved, including workers' compensation insurers, workers' compensation administrative agencies, or employers who are coordinating the coverage of medical costs and partial wages. These agencies may request and be granted access to relevant medical records, such as evaluation results. What this means is that if you receive care through workers' compensation, you may not have the right to privacy of your medical records.

If you have questions or concerns about your privacy when applying for workers' compensation, it may be helpful to arrange a meeting with your employer's privacy office, attorney, or case manager to obtain more information.

Summary

This chapter discussed some of the specific considerations for an employee who sustains a concussion. Generally speaking, if you have sustained a concussion, you should try to get back to your typical work routine as soon as you can unless your work involves potentially dangerous activities. This may be challenging if your symptoms interfere with your ability to safely complete work tasks or to be productive while at work. In addition, work settings may make your concussion symptoms worse, and, as a result, taking medical leave for some length of time may be warranted. It is crucial that you maintain an open dialogue with your health care providers and employer following a concussion to promote a smooth transition back to work.

Military Concussions

In this chapter, you will learn:

- Special considerations related to concussion in military personnel and associated challenges
- Common conditions that accompany military concussion
- How military concussions are acutely managed
- How return-to-duty decisions are made

In this chapter we will discuss some of the unique considerations associated with concussions in military personnel, as well as specialized considerations related to treatment and return to duty. For military personnel, military health care providers will provide the important care described in the early chapters of this book, including urgent evaluation after suspected concussion, removal from dangerous activities and further evaluation if needed, and close monitoring during recovery. Military health care providers will also provide education on what to expect with symptoms and recovery. If you are a service member who has persisting symptoms after concussion, you will likely undergo more comprehensive evaluation. The goal of this chapter is to help you understand the special circumstances and considerations related to concussions in military personnel.

Military concussions are common and have become increasingly prevalent in recent years with the increased use of improvised explosive devices (IEDs) in warfare. IEDs are homemade bombs that cause explosive force that is often transmitted to the brain, resulting in concussion, or can throw military service members to the ground or against structures, resulting in head impacts. Sophisticated advances in helmets and body armor technology have helped military personnel survive injuries that would previously have been fatal, and although more military personnel survive serious injuries, they often survive with other injuries, including traumatic brain injury (TBI). While head impacts may result in moderate to severe TBI, concussion is the most common type of brain injury. Concussions that affect military personnel tend to be associated with other medical and psychological conditions that can affect aspects of recovery and return to duty or combat. It is important to realize that military concussions can occur while military personnel are serving at their home base or can occur in the military theater during deployment to a combat zone. This chapter discusses some of the common mechanisms of injury and some unique considerations for military personnel across a variety of settings.

Mechanisms of Military Concussion

The majority of concussions in military personnel are not deployment-related, meaning they do not occur in combat but happen during military training or participation in sports or in motor vehicle collisions. In these cases, concussive injuries result from **blunt head trauma**, such as from a fall or a hit to the head. They may result from the rapid acceleration and deceleration that occurs in motor vehicle collisions, whether occurring during military service activities or when off duty. These types of concussions experienced by service members are quite similar to those experienced by civilians, and thus recommendations for evaluating these concussions are generally the same as we discussed earlier in the book.

Military personnel may also experience injuries from being near a large explosion. Explosions generate blast energy and can cause a specific type of injury called a blast injury (see also Chapter 1). When explosives detonate, a wave of high pressure compresses the air, resulting in negative pressure that then displaces air, causing a **blast wave**. The blast wave can transmit force to the brain, causing a concussion or a more severe form of TBI. Blast waves can produce brain dysfunction in several different ways. They can directly disrupt brain tissue, which is called a **primary injury**. A **secondary injury** can occur when the blast displaces shrapnel or other objects at high speeds, which can then hit a person's head or even penetrate the skull. A third injury—or **tertiary injury**—can occur when the explosion results in the service member being thrown to the ground or against another stationary object at high speed. Finally, a **quaternary injury** may occur when a person is exposed to chemical toxins, thermal energy, or radiation that may be released during an explosion. Primary, secondary, and tertiary injury mechanisms are illustrated in Figure 14.1. Blast injuries involve a variety of complex changes within the body, and we are still learning about the exact ways they affect the brain's functioning. Understanding the effects of primary blast injury

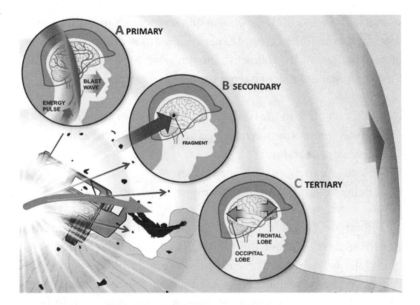

FIGURE 14.1. Blast injury modalities

Originally published in James Singleton and Jon Clasper. "Trauma in Conflict Zones" in Oxford Textbook of Fundamentals of Surgery Copyright © 2016, Oxford Publishing Limited. DOI: 10.1093/med/9780199665549.003.0093. Reproduced with permission of Oxford Publishing Limited through PLSclear.

combined with a penetrating or blunt injury from the same incident (sometimes referred to as "blast-plus") can be particularly challenging. Blast injuries and other forms of military concussion may also be associated with other medical and psychological conditions that can make recovery more complex and challenging.

Screening for and Management of Military Concussion

A variety of protocols are in place to ensure the safety of military personnel suspected of injury during deployment. First, whenever possible, any individuals experiencing concussion-related symptoms will be removed from combat until they have fully recovered, thereby protecting them from recurrent injury. Furthermore, military personnel will need to undergo concussion screening and 24-hour mandated rest, even if they are not experiencing any symptoms, if they are involved in any of the following situations while deployed for which there is a potential risk of having sustained a concussion:

- A direct blow to the head or episode of loss of consciousness
- Involvement in any vehicle accident that results in a blast, collision, or rollover
- Exposure to more than one blast event
- Being within 50 meters of a known explosion

Military concussion is managed in accordance with standard guidelines developed for the military from initial screening to specialty follow-up. Immediately after a suspected military concussion, injured personnel will be evaluated by a medic or corpsman at a battalion aid station. The medic or corpsman will gather information about the injury and associated symptoms and perform a brief standardized neurologic examination. If any red flags or concerns are discovered during this brief evaluation, the injured service member may be taken to an in-theater concussion care center, where a physician and occupational therapy technician can conduct cognitive testing to obtain objective information about how the injured service member's brain is functioning. Based on that evaluation, the service member may begin a 2-week rehabilitation program designed to help them get back on track. Military treatment providers provide a targeted symptom approach to treat symptoms of concussion using treatments similar to those described in earlier chapters.

If the results are concerning or abnormal in any way, the service member may be taken to an infield hospital for specialty care procedures, such as neuroimaging, to rule out a more serious brain injury that would require additional interventions. Military personnel who require further medical intervention at this point (for example, those who have positive neuroimaging findings indicating a more severe form of TBI), are relocated to a hospital facility for stabilization until they can be transported to a Department of Defense military hospital in Europe or the United States.

Returning to Duty after a Concussion

As with screening procedures, military **return-to-duty** procedures after a concussion are carried out in a standard fashion in accordance with specific guidelines. Reliable standardization of these guidelines is critical because a recently concussed soldier returning to combat too soon may put their own life and the lives of others at risk. The return-to-duty evaluation begins when the service member has recovered to the point where they have no symptoms at rest, whether with or without treatment. As with athletes who have sustained a concussion while playing a sport, active-duty personnel who are injured in the military theater must be free of impairing symptoms both while at rest and with both mental and physical exertion before returning to full duty. A return-to-duty evaluation includes observing the service member while they are undergoing exertion to see whether exertion provokes any symptoms. Military personnel with any active concussion symptoms are not allowed to resume full duties until they are cleared by medical personnel.

Computerized cognitive testing is used to measure aspects of thinking skills that are often affected by concussion. These same tests are first administered at baseline before the military person is deployed so that any concussion-related changes can be detected. Changes in testing performance from baseline to post-concussion are then used to guide decisions about return to duty. If the concussed military service member is not yet performing at their baseline, it is probably not safe for them to resume their full in-theater military duties. It is important to note that any small persisting symptoms can have very serious consequences in the context of a demanding combat-related situation. To keep all military service members safe, it is very important to make sure that anyone who has a concussion has fully recovered before they resume full service activities.

Conditions That May Accompany Military Concussion

Given that service members may experience concussions during combat or from explosions in the military theater, they may experience multiple other injuries, including serious damage to limbs and/or internal organs, as well as psychological trauma.

Polytrauma

Blast injuries often result in damage to multiple body parts and organ systems, a phenomenon that is referred to as **polytrauma**. One of the most common forms of polytrauma involves damage to the body's hearing and visual systems. Research has shown that hearing loss is extremely common among veterans who were involved in military conflicts in which IEDs were commonly used. Hearing problems can result from a number of causes, including rupture of the eardrum (**tympanic membrane**). Blast injuries may also rupture structures within the eye, although these types of visual system disturbances are more common in moderate to severe blast-related injuries. Significant blast pressure and associated injury mechanisms can also cause damage to the lungs (blast lung) and abdominal organs (blast belly), resulting in a host of associated challenges. Polytrauma due to blast injury may also include spinal cord injury, burn injuries, and badly injured arms or legs which may require amputation. Individuals with polytrauma require coordinated care from an interdisciplinary medical team that can collectively address all aspects of the injury. Medical stabilization and rehabilitation of evolving physical injuries may take precedence over concussion management in these situations. In short, saving the life of injured personnel is the top priority; less severe injuries may not be evaluated or diagnosed when life-threatening injuries occur. Typically, service members with serious bodily injuries are evacuated to a military hospital outside of the active combat zone. Once there, they are routinely screened for concussion. This is done to ensure that a concussion is not overshadowed by other injuries and that, if diagnosed, concussion can be managed as part of their overall treatment plan.

Jared was medically discharged from the U.S. Army after sustaining a mild TBI, among other significant injuries, secondary to a car bomb explosion during his deployment in Iraq. Jared lost a battalion mate in the accident and experienced posttraumatic stress symptoms, including flashbacks and nightmares about the event. Upon returning home, Jared has a hard time keeping a job and starts to struggle in his relationships. He is restless at night and starts drinking alcohol to fall asleep. He is able to see a therapist at the Department of Veterans Affairs hospital, who works with him to get on a daily routine that involves significant exercise and regular sleep and wake times. Jared works with the therapist to develop organizational strategies that become really helpful as he applies for jobs. After about 6 weeks, Jared is getting into a better routine, and his relationships are improving. He is feeling less scattered and more in control of his thoughts and emotions. Eventually, he and his therapist are able to address the trauma he experienced, and his flashbacks and nightmares become less frequent and less impairing in his day-to-day life.

Psychological Comorbidities

Service members who sustain a concussion in combat also have an increased risk for various accompanying psychological problems based on the body's response to the injury. Some of the same brain networks that are important for managing stress and anxiety may be affected directly by injury. Research has shown that a large number of individuals who have experienced a combat injury may experience symptoms of acute stress or symptoms commonly associated with posttraumatic stress disorder (PTSD; see also Chapter 4). Within the military, these symptoms are referred to as posttraumatic stress. Some of these symptoms may overlap with symptoms experienced following a concussion. The most effective management plans acknowledge and incorporate the symptoms of both concussion and posttraumatic stress, rather than solely focusing on one or the other. Posttraumatic stress can cause several different problems that occur during the day, including being hypervigilant to one's surroundings; experiencing flashbacks; feeling emotionally numb; and avoiding certain activities, places, or people. Posttraumatic stress also typically involves nighttime difficulties, such as nightmares and reduced sleep quality. If you are a military service member and think you may have symptoms of posttraumatic stress in addition to a concussion, it is important to communicate this information to your health care team. Posttraumatic stress is treatable and is not something that anyone needs to "power through" or try to ignore. Although medications such as selective serotonin reuptake inhibitors (SSRIs) or prazosin, which can target nightmares, can be helpful in managing symptoms of posttraumatic stress, behavioral treatments that do not involve medications, such as exposure therapy, cognitive processing therapy, and **eye movement desensitization and reprocessing (EMDR)**, can be extremely helpful. If an injured loved one experiences a potentially traumatic event, you should encourage them to fully disclose any and all symptoms to their health care team so the team can provide the best care to ensure their health and recovery.

Summary

This chapter discussed the common mechanisms of military concussion, some of the unique challenges military personnel may experience with a concussion, the process in which military personnel are screened for a concussion in theater, and how military concussions are managed. As with athletes who sustain a suspected concussion while playing a sport, military personnel need to be promptly removed from the combat situation and carefully evaluated. Standardized protocols are then used to rule out more severe injuries and to ensure a safe return to duty. Any associated symptoms, such as polytrauma or posttraumatic stress, should be incorporated into a comprehensive treatment plan.

Concussions in Older Adults

In this chapter, you will learn:

- Risk factors for concussion in older adults
- Common conditions that may accompany or complicate concussion recovery in older adults
- Special considerations for concussion diagnosis and management in older adults

As we age, physical changes occur within our bodies and brains that increase the risk of concussion and more severe forms of brain injury and can make recovery more difficult. Due to these age-related changes in the brain, older adults are more likely to experience complications and prolonged recovery after head injury. Over time, the brain starts to shrink, resulting in decreased brain volume and weight, a phenomenon called **brain atrophy**. In addition, with aging comes a reduction in **neural plasticity**, the brain's ability to make new connections and adapt to changes following an injury. Older adults are at increased risk of having a brain bleed following a head injury, particularly those who are on **anticoagulant medications** or medications that thin the blood (commonly called blood thinners). For this reason, CT scans and MRI scans are frequently performed in older patients with suspected head injuries. If you are an older adult, brain imaging is an important consideration in the acute assessment of head injuries to rule out a more serious injury.

Research has shown that older adults are more likely than younger individuals to experience physical and cognitive difficulties following a brain injury, although this is more typical in cases of moderate to severe traumatic brain injury than in concussion. Generally speaking, if you are an older adult, your recovery will likely take longer after concussion. Having other medical conditions may also complicate your recovery. It is important for you to be patient and maintain a positive perspective.

Mary is an 83-year-old retired librarian with diabetes, high blood pressure, and arthritis who lives alone. Mary is able to walk short distances using a cane and drives herself to her local community center to swim laps 1 day each week. Mary is leaving the pool after swimming laps one day when her vision becomes blurry and she loses her footing and falls to the ground. Mary feels very fatigued and cannot get up without help. Paramedics take her to the hospital, where an evaluation indicates that Mary's blood sugar level has dropped too low. A brain scan does not show any abnormalities, and Mary is discharged from the hospital with instructions to rest her hip, which has been badly bruised. A few days later, Mary gets lost while driving to her chiropractor's office. She pulls over and calls her daughter, who helps her to remain calm and find her way back to a familiar location. Mary's daughter is worried that her mother might have sustained a concussion during her fall and schedules an appointment for Mary to be seen at a specialty concussion clinic. Upon evaluation, Mary shares that she had gotten lost while driving several times in the past 6 months, something that she had not shared with her daughter until this most recent occasion. Results of the evaluation suggest that Mary's difficulties are not caused by concussion but by her other medical conditions and early signs of dementia. Mary is provided with some tools to help her manage her existing health conditions and cognitive symptoms. She is encouraged to follow up with a neurologist who specializes in the assessment and treatment of aging-related brain changes. Upon evaluation, the neurologist tells Mary that it was important that she had a brain scan after her fall to rule out an acute brain bleed. He also tells her that he is glad that the specialty concussion clinic realized that many of her symptoms started before the concussion and referred her for further neuro-logic evaluation.

Risk Factors for Concussion in the Older Adult

The most common cause of concussion in older adults is falls, which can occur for a number of reasons. In fact, when an older adult sustains a concussion due to a fall, it becomes important not only to treat the person for any fall-related injuries but also to check for underlying conditions that might have led to the fall in the first place. If you are an older adult, you might fall while walking on a slippery surface or because you have **arthritis** pain that makes it difficult for you to sufficiently pick up your feet. Laboratory testing might indicate that you had a fall because of acute **hypoglycemia**, a condition that arises when blood sugar levels drop too low. Low blood sugar levels can result in fatigue and visual disturbance as well as other symptoms. Many underlying conditions and situations have been shown to increase an older adult's risk for falling or being involved in an accident:

- Medical conditions
  - Neurologic problems (e.g., stroke, Parkinson's disease, dementia)
  - Visual disturbances (e.g., **cataracts, glaucoma**)
  - Musculoskeletal problems (e.g., arthritis)
  - Acute conditions (e.g., **postural hypotension**, substance use, medication effects)
- Aging-related conditions
  - Decreased reaction time, which can lead to motor vehicle accidents

- o Slowed walking pace, which can lead to pedestrian accidents
- Environmental conditions
  - o Insufficient lighting
  - o Slippery walking surfaces
  - o Poor traction in shoes or ill-fitting shoes
- Activity-related conditions
  - o Walking down stairs
  - o Climbing ladders or stairs
  - o Participating in recreational activities (e.g., cycling or pickleball)

It is important to note that many of the same factors that may predispose you to falls as an older adult also increase your risk of being involved in motor vehicle or other accidents. For example, if you cannot see clearly, you may be more likely to trip on an object and also more likely to get into a traffic accident.

Another cause of concussion among older adults is assault. Older individuals are at an increased risk of physical, verbal, and other types of abuse, such as neglect. This is particularly true among older adults lacking strong family and social support. For this reason, older adults being evaluated for a suspected brain injury are usually asked to complete an elder abuse or elder mistreatment screening measure, a questionnaire that helps providers identify signs of elder abuse. Your health care providers will want to intervene to help you and get appropriate resources if they believe that you have been or are being abused.

Concussion Assessment and Management in Older Adults

Following evaluation in the Emergency Room where brain imaging is typically done to rule out a brain bleed, further evaluation and management are conducted in an outpatient clinic setting. When evaluating a person with a suspected concussion, a key component to the diagnosis involves understanding what the person was like before the injury. This becomes increasingly important when assessing older adults, who are more likely to have other health conditions that may contribute to signs and symptoms of concussion. In addition, aging can cause changes to thinking abilities and physical functioning that may be present before a suspected injury. If you are injured and suspect that you might have sustained a concussion, it is important to bring someone who knows you well or spends a lot of time with you, such as a family member or close friend, to your medical appointments. This friend or family member will be asked to provide information about what you were like before your injury.

As part of the evaluation for concussion, you will also have a physical examination. Your health care provider will ask questions about your current symptoms, any symptoms you had before your injury, other diagnosed health conditions, and the medications you take. It can be very helpful to bring a list of your medications to this appointment, especially if you take a lot of different medications. Your health care team will also want to know how independent you are in carrying out activities of daily living. Do you take care of everything yourself or do you need others to help you with your daily activities? In addition, your health care provider may conduct a brief cognitive assessment to learn about your current thinking abilities.

In some cases, you may be referred to a neuropsychologist for more in-depth assessment of your thinking skills. Neuropsychologists conduct testing that can help determine the cause of cognitive concerns and identify the most appropriate course for treatment. In many cases, cognitive difficulties in older adults stem from a variety of factors (as seen in the case example) and may have been present before a suspected concussion. A large portion of adults over the age of 85 are affected by either dementia (a loss in cognitive functioning that makes it difficult for a person to carry out daily tasks and maintain independence) or **mild cognitive impairment** (a loss of cognitive performance that is not yet severe enough to cause impairments in daily function). Although many of the cognitive symptoms of concussion overlap with those of dementia, the symptoms of dementia are more chronic and do not get better with time. Alzheimer's dementia is the most common form of dementia, affecting memory, language, and executive functions. Many other forms of dementia exist, including **vascular dementia**, a condition that results from multiple silent strokes and can produce a wide variety of cognitive problems, such as reduced executive functions (multitasking) and processing speed (slower thinking). Alzheimer's disease and vascular dementia frequently occur together and are the two most common forms of dementia. It is not unusual for early signs of dementia to go unnoticed because these symptoms may be incorrectly chalked up to normal aging. In addition, older adults experiencing cognitive changes, such as memory lapses, may develop compensatory strategies over time. It is important to realize that a concussion can temporarily make it more difficult for an older adult to use existing compensatory strategies, making the impact of a concussive injury appear more severe. In some cases, the difficulty with compensatory strategies produced by a concussion can unmask previously unidentified mild cognitive impairment or early dementia. Based on the patterns and results that can be determined by expert interpretation of neuropsychological testing, accurate information can be obtained helping to identify if there were underlying cognitive issues that existed prior to the injury that may be contributing to the current challenges following concussion due to either the loss of ability to compensate or whether other injury symptoms may be affecting cognitive performance.

Common Comorbidities and Other Factors Affecting Recovery

If you are older and your concussion occurred as a result of a fall or other accident, you may have also injured other parts of your body, which may further complicate recovery. Bone fractures are very common, which can make it difficult for you to get around without assistance. Falls and other injuries are also likely to result in bruising, or **contusions**, which can be painful and reduce mobility. Unfortunately, a loss of mobility can decrease your independence, which may be a huge adjustment from what you were used to before your injury. Furthermore, decreased mobility can make it significantly more difficult for you to get out and spend time with your loved ones, which is an important part of recovery.

As an older adult, you may also have preexisting chronic pain that may make recovery more difficult following a concussion. Examples of preexisting pain conditions include **neuropathic pain**, a common complication of diabetes, and pain from arthritis, a condition that causes painful inflammation within the joints. Pain can make it more challenging to concentrate and solve problems, making tasks such as driving more difficult and even unsafe. In addition, pain can make it more difficult to fall asleep or stay asleep and has been linked with emotional problems, such as depression and anxiety. It is very important to discuss any pain you may have with your health care provider so that your pain level can be appropriately managed.

Another important consideration for you as an older adult with a concussion is related to your use of medications. Many older individuals take a variety of medications for management of chronic health conditions. In fact, research suggests that over half of individuals over the age of 65 take five or more medications each day. These medications may interact with one another and with any new medications your health care provider may prescribe following a concussion. It is important to talk openly with your health care provider about any medications that you are taking. If possible, it is best to bring a list of your current medications and their dosages to any medical appointments. The list should include any over-the-counter medications and supplements you take.

It is important for the doctors managing your concussion to be aware of all your medications to help them better understand your preexisting medical conditions, make better treatment decisions for your concussion symptoms, and avoid drug combinations that could cause side effects. Also, it is helpful to use only one pharmacy so your **pharmacist** can take an extra look at any medications you are taking to further ensure that no potential for dangerous interactions between medications exists. If you are an older adult who has sustained a concussion, it is important that you not use any over-the-counter medications without first consulting with your health care provider or a pharmacist. This is because older adults process and clear medications from the body differently than younger adults. Some over-the-counter medications are sedating or cause cognitive difficulties in older adults and could further complicate recovery after concussion.

Concussion and Aging

A variety of treatments are available to help older adults who have been diagnosed with a concussion after other common causes of persisting cognitive symptoms have been ruled out. Many of these interventions are aimed at reducing the effects of pain, sleep disturbance, and mood problems, all of which tend to have a negative impact on thinking skills. Many of the therapies described in Chapter 8 of this book, including cognitive-behavioral therapy, can be extremely helpful strategies for managing pain, increasing sleep quality, and improving mood following a concussion. If evaluation identifies a suspicion of underlying mild cognitive impairment, then your provider may incorporate a medication such as a cholinesterase inhibitor or memantine meant to slow memory decline as discussed in Chapter 8. In addition, therapy with a psychologist or occupational therapist can help you learn strategies to cope with or work around cognitive problems you might be experiencing. For example, if you are having memory problems, your psychologist or therapist might help you develop compensatory strategies such as writing down important information in a notebook or

TABLE 15.1 Cognitive Concerns and Compensatory Strategies

Thinking Concern	Strategy or Resource
Attention/multitasking	• Focus on one task at a time; avoid multitasking. • If you have a big project, focus on one small step at a time. • Face people when talking and make eye contact to improve focus. • Ask people to summarize key points of their conversation with you. You can ask them for a take-home message. • Put important items such as your keys, wallet, and glasses in the same place every day, such as in a special basket or bowl, so you are less likely to misplace them. • Reduce distractions when you are reading; turn off the television or music. It may help to follow along with your finger and stop after each paragraph to think about the most important point.
Forgetfulness for medications	• Use a pillbox for your medications. Fill up the pillbox once a week or have someone else fill it for you or check to make sure you did it correctly. Using a pillbox reduces the chance you'll miss doses or accidentally take too much medicine. • Set an alarm on your phone, watch, or clock to remind you to take your medications. • Use a smartphone app to help you remember to take your medications. • If it works with your medications, try using a mail-order pharmacy service to make it easier to take your medications as prescribed. • As long as you do not have young children in your home, put your medications next to your toothbrush as a visual cue to remind you to take them.

(continued)

TABLE 15.1 Continued

Thinking Concern	Strategy or Resource
Memory	• Keep a small notebook with you to write down important information, or use the notes function on your smartphone. • Put sticky notes with reminders where you will see them, such as on your bathroom mirror or the interior of your front door. • Keep important information in a three-ring binder so you can find it when you need it. • Keep a list of important phone numbers next to your phone. • Use a large calendar or whiteboard in your kitchen to keep appointments and other important information visible.
Slowed thinking	• Ask people to slow down when they talk to you. • Take your time when you are completing tasks and take short breaks. • Allow yourself extra time so you do not feel rushed; it is okay to take longer to complete tasks.

calendar. Table 15.1 lists examples of common cognitive concerns after concussion in older adults and specific strategies to help compensate for each type of concern. In some cases, your doctor may recommend that you make changes to your diet or increase your daily exercise, which have been shown to improve thinking skills in both older and younger adults. If you are an older adult, it is important to remember that your recovery after concussion may be slower than younger adults, but these tips and strategies may help you during your recovery.

Summary

This chapter provided information about common causes of concussion in older adults and factors that may affect recovery after concussion. If you are an older adult with a concussion, be sure to talk to your health care provider about any other medical conditions you have and bring a list of all medications you are currently taking. Whenever possible, it is best for you to bring a family member or close friend with you to your medical appointment so they can provide the doctor with information about what you were like before the injury and how you are doing now. Taking these steps will help ensure that you get the best care possible during recovery.

Section 4

Conclusion and What's Next

Where Have We Been and Where Are We Going?

In this chapter, you will learn:

- How increased public awareness about concussion has led to safety initiatives
- How research has changed best practices for concussion care
- About innovations in technology for diagnosing and managing concussion
- Areas for future research

One of the biggest challenges with concussion is that it is considered an invisible injury. Someone who is experiencing symptoms of a concussion may not show obvious outward signs of trauma such as they would with a broken bone. While the injury may be invisible to others, a concussion can cause significant impairment in your daily functioning and you may experience frustration that others do not understand what you are going through.

Fortunately, public knowledge around the importance of concussion and its associated symptoms has increased dramatically in the recent past. Many people now have a greater appreciation for some of the challenges associated with concussion and may be more understanding if you are struggling in the early days after your injury or if you have persisting symptoms after concussion. This heightened public awareness has led all 50 states to implement guidelines for the acute management of concussions in public high schools, promote training designed to increase awareness (and thus improve diagnosis), and introduce appropriate measures such as a gradual return to learning and sports. The military has also developed a more extensive screening program to evaluate for concussions and manage recovery and promote a safe return to duty. Public safety campaigns have emphasized the importance of wearing helmets during recreational activity such as cycling, skiing, and snowboarding, and many nursing homes and assisted living facilities have implemented fall prevention programs to reduce the risk of head injury. Work is continuing on these public health initiatives focusing on increasing awareness and safety.

While there are intriguing advances in technology on the horizon for the evaluation and management of concussion, research continues to demonstrate that simple education about concussion is one of the most important factors to shorten the recovery period and improve outcome. It can be very distressing to experience the symptoms of concussion and to worry about what lies ahead. Learning about concussion recovery and what to expect can set positive and realistic expectations for your recovery. We as clinicians and researchers have learned a lot about concussion over the past several years. Based on clinical research, more health care providers now understand the importance of promoting an earlier, gradual return to activity to promote recovery.

Health care providers now have access to a variety of research-based clinical tools and questionnaires that allow for identification of all symptoms that may be associated with a concussion, including physical symptoms (headaches, dizziness, and sleep dysfunction), emotional symptoms (irritability, anxiety, depression), and cognitive symptoms (impairments in attention, concentration, and memory). If you are not recovering as expected or your symptoms are persisting, comprehensive assessment allows health care providers to develop a more tailored management plan to help you recover. This tailored management plan may involve a variety of different health care providers with specialized expertise in one or more of these symptoms. Having a systematic approach helps health care providers determine when other professionals may be needed to help with your overall recovery plan.

Advancing Technology

Interest in the use of technology to further improve the detection and management of concussion is growing. Advances have been made in event detection (identifying when a concussion has occurred), clinical diagnostic assessments, and biomarkers.

Event detection technology has its best potential application in military and sports-related concussions and includes technology such as helmet sensors and body sensors. This type of technology may help identify significant forces being transmitted to the brain before concussion symptoms are observed. Being able to detect excess forces affecting the brain before a clinically observable injury—a concussion diagnosis—may help make military service and contact sports safer. This technology may also provide information about subconcussive events (impacts that do not cause observable clinical signs or symptoms) and how these events may relate to the future development of clinical problems. New technology in clinical diagnostic assessment of concussion symptoms includes sophisticated equipment for measuring and evaluating eye movements and for evaluating posture and balance.

A great deal of research has been conducted on biomarkers to help detect whether a concussion has occurred. These biomarkers include proteins in blood or spinal fluid, imaging markers using more advanced analysis techniques or neurophysiological measurements such as brain waves (EEG), and variability in heart rate. To date, most research on these biomarkers has focused on confirming the diagnosis of concussion. It is hoped that future research can help identify practical biomarkers for concussion and more severe forms of brain injury that can guide rehabilitation and provide clinical information about recovery expectations.

Challenging Questions for the Future

We are still trying to learn why some individuals who have a concussion do well and recover quickly, whereas others may have more severe symptoms or a longer recovery period. Biology and genetics may contribute to differences in concussion risk and recovery. In addition, personality variables, positive mindset, and coping skills may also be factors. In fact, the military has developed trainings around these positive psychological and behavioral skills to improve the resilience of military personnel. If we can learn more about how and why some people have better outcomes, we hope to be able to use this information to facilitate recovery in a greater number of people.

We are still trying to understand why some individuals with numerous recurrent concussions or subconcussive injury develop later complications, such as chronic traumatic encephalopathy (see Chapter 9). In particular, scientists are working to understand how concerning changes in the brain can be detected early and in people who are still alive. It is likely that some people have a greater susceptibility to a poor outcome; understanding these individual differences will be important in helping everyone make informed decisions about participating in activities that may increase their risk. New technologies, such as blood or spinal fluid biomarkers and advances in imaging techniques, may ultimately provide more specific information about future risk that can help with making these important personal decisions about participating in activities with an elevated risk of concussion or subconcussive injury.

As science advances, more challenging management questions may arise. As we learn more about who is at greater risk for poor outcome after concussion based on genetics or other factors, should this information affect who plays contact sports? That will be an important and complex ethical question for health care and our society in general.

Currently, the clinical indicator for full clearance to return to work, school, or sport is resolution of clinical symptoms that are not made worse by activity. As new biomarkers emerge and new technologies advance, we will need to figure out what to do when someone is symptom-free after their concussion, but they continue to have an abnormal biomarker or other indicator of incomplete recovery. Should a biomarker without observable clinical symptoms be a limiting factor on clearance and return to typical activities? These advances may also help us better understand how someone responds to treatments or rehabilitation after concussion. Hopefully these new technologies may also provide data on what interventions might enhance recovery after concussion and which interventions are no more effective than natural recovery.

Summary

Many advancements have occurred and controversies arisen around concussion over the past several years. Even after years of scientific research, we continue to look for even more answers to keep people safe and healthy. Most health care providers and researchers have the same goal: to allow people to live their lives to the fullest, participate in activities they enjoy, prevent injury as much as possible, and, when a concussion occurs, help them recover as smoothly as possible and get back to living their life. A lot has been learned about concussion over the years, and we are excited for what the future holds as advances in technology and research bring us to the next generation of concussion care.

Conclusion

This book has covered a lot of information about concussion. In the first section, you learned that a concussion is a temporary disruption in the brain's normal functioning caused by traumatic force to the brain or body. This disruption in brain function affects the brain's ability to process information, resulting in either an alteration in consciousness or, more rarely, a loss of consciousness.

A concussion is different than many other brain conditions because it typically does not involve structural damage to brain cells that can be seen on standard imaging. Accurate detection and diagnosis of a concussion is challenging because brain scans, such as CT or MRI, are designed to look for structural damage. If you received a head CT or brain MRI, it was used to rule out a more serious brain injury.

In the first days to weeks after injury, concussion can present in a number of ways to include physical, cognitive, or emotional symptoms. Because of the variety of symptoms, it is important that you see a health care provider who can evaluate your specific symptoms. Not everyone has all the possible symptoms of concussion, and your symptoms may be different than the symptoms experienced by a friend or neighbor who has had a concussion. Most people with concussion begin recovering within days to weeks and will start to feel more like themselves again.

Your safety is a primary concern after concussion. Given that your brain is still vulnerable while recovering from a concussion, your health care provider will want to reduce your risk of further injury. This may mean keeping an athlete on the sidelines or limiting work for someone whose job may have potential for injury. If you have severe symptoms during the early days after concussion, your health care provider may offer treatment options such as pain relievers for headache and provide you with recommendations for managing school or work.

Head injuries have been recognized as an important area of medicine for a long time. Hippocrates, the father of modern medicine, observed, "No head injury is too trivial to ignore." Those words continue to be true today. Our understanding of concussion has continued to grow even in the past 10 to 20 years, and exciting research is under way to learn more about persisting symptoms and long-term complications.

A multidisciplinary approach to concussion management really is a team approach, and the most important member of any treatment team is you. Understanding how a concussion affects you and your family is an important part of creating a treatment plan that can be individualized and tailored to you. Now that you know more about concussion and what to expect, we hope you can successfully navigate the challenges of concussion. Thank you for allowing us to be part of your journey.

GLOSSARY

504 plan: plan that outlines formal academic adjustments/accommodations to provide individualized support for students with learning problems, concentration difficulties, intellectual disability, and a host of other conditions who may require extra support in an academic environment.

Acceleration–deceleration injury: specific type of brain injury that results from rapid acceleration (or speeding up) followed by rapid deceleration (or slowing down).

Activity pacing: component of certain psychological and physical therapy treatments that involves tracking pain levels and learning to identify patterns in pain to avoid pain flare-ups and improve overall functioning.

Acute posttraumatic headaches: headaches that develop within 7 days of a head injury; also called post-concussive headaches.

Acute stress disorder: trauma-related disorder in which the individual has symptoms of posttraumatic stress disorder (PTSD) but not much time has passed since the traumatic exposure (between 3 days and 1 month).

Advanced practice nurse: nurse with master's-level or doctoral-level training who can diagnose and prescribe treatments independently or in collaboration with a physician.

Alzheimer's dementia: the most common form of dementia; can affect memory, language, and/or executive functioning skills, resulting in impaired functional abilities and independence.

Amyotrophic lateral sclerosis (ALS): a neurologic condition which results in progressive weakness in the arms and legs as well as muscles used for talking and swallowing.

Anhedonia: inability to experience positive emotions.

Anticoagulant medications: medications used to treat and prevent blood clots; sometimes referred to as blood thinners.

Antidepressant medication: type of medication used to treat depression and other mood disorders as well as other mental and physical illnesses.

Antihypertensives: medications used to control blood pressure.

Antiseizure medications: medications used to control and prevent the onset of seizures; also called antiepileptic drugs (AEDs).

Anxiety: excessive worry that is difficult to control.

Apo e4: a version of the apolipoprotein E gene that is associated with Alzheimer's disease.

Arthritis: condition that causes painful inflammation within the joints.

Athletic trainer: skilled professional who has extensive training in working with other health care professionals to identify and manage injuries that occur in sports.

Attention-deficit/hyperactivity disorder (ADHD): a condition that is present in childhood that results in attention, concentration, and/or hyperactive and impulsive symptoms that cause interference in daily functioning across settings or environments.

Atypical neuroleptic medication: class of medications often used to treat psychiatric conditions because of their action on certain neurotransmitters (chemicals within the brain).

Autonomic arousal: activation of the body's "fight-or-flight" system that increases heart rate and blood pressure.

Autonomic dysfunction: disruption within the body's system that regulates unconscious functions such as heart rate and blood pressure.

Axons: parts of brain cells that help transmit information from one brain cell to another.

Balance Error Scoring System (BESS): objective balance assessment that requires patients to stand in a variety of positions.

Behavior: way in which a person or animal acts or behaves.

Behavioral activation: form of behavioral therapy that involves increasing one's level of daily activities to improve emotional functioning.

Benign paroxysmal positional vertigo (BPPV): condition that causes episodes of vertigo that are triggered with head movements.

Biochemical changes: changes to the chemical processes within living things.

Biofeedback: a type of treatment that uses sensors that measure muscle tension, heart rate, or skin temperature to provide feedback about the body's response to stress and how to manage and reduce the stress response.

Biomarkers: markers in the blood or saliva or other bodily tissues that help medical providers diagnose certain conditions or monitor aspects of recovery.

Biomechanical forces: mechanical forces related to the human body.

Blast injuries: injuries that can occur as a result of forces produced after an explosion.

Blast wave: wave of high pressure that compresses air and results in negative pressure that then displaces air after an explosive detonates.

Blunt head trauma: trauma that may result from hitting one's head against an object or the ground.

Botulinum toxin (Botox): treatment for chronic migraines; injection of botulinum toxin into the muscles of the head has been shown to have a therapeutic effect.

Brain atrophy: shrinkage of the brain over time as a result of healthy aging or neurodegenerative disease or injury.

Brain-derived neurotrophic factor (BDNF): protein that helps support brain cells and their connections.

Brain fibers: parts of brain cells that transmit information from one brain cell to another; also called axons.

Brain injury: insult to the brain; can be traumatic or acquired via other causes, such as stroke or tumor.

Brainstem: the most inferior part of the brain; it extends into the spinal cord and plays an important role in maintaining vital functions, including breathing.

Calcitonin-gene related peptide (CGRP): inflammatory protein thought to play a role in headache pain.

Calcitonin gene-related peptide receptor antagonists: new class of medications that show promise in treating migraine; also called CGRP inhibitors.

Cataracts: medical condition in which the lens of the eye becomes more and more opaque over time, causing blurred vision.

Catch-up saccades: abnormal eye movements that can occur when the head is thrust in different directions during evaluation or when damage to the neurovisual system has occurred; also called nystagmus.

Central: when used in a medical context, referring to the central nervous system (within the brain and/or spinal cord).

Certified athletic trainer: skilled professional who has extensive training in working with other health care professionals to identify and manage injuries that occur in sports.

Cervicalgia: pain that starts along the cervical spine at the neck or upper shoulders and often causes headaches.

Cervicogenic headache: headache caused by changes within the cervical spine.

CGRP: calcitonin gene-related peptide; thought to play a role in headache pain.

CGRP inhibitors: new class of medications that show promise in treating migraine; also called calcitonin gene-related peptide receptor antagonists.

Cholinesterase inhibitor: medication that blocks the breakdown of acetylcholine which is most commonly used in the management of dementia.

Chronic posttraumatic headaches: headaches that continue for 3 months or longer after a concussion.

Chronic traumatic encephalopathy (CTE): neuropathologic condition that is diagnosed at autopsy based upon a signature of proteins that aggregate within the brain and is thought to be associated with chronic subconcussive head injuries over an extended period of time.

Cocooning: colloquialism used to describe outdated concussion management recommendations involving rest in a dark space and avoidance of all activities.

Cognitive-behavioral therapy (CBT): psychological treatment that teaches patients how to identify negative thoughts and arrive at more balanced thoughts as well as understand the relationship between thoughts, emotions, and behaviors.

Cognitive-behavioral therapy for insomnia (CBTi): psychological treatment that works to relieve problems with falling or staying asleep through a variety of techniques that improve sleep quality.

Cognitive deconditioning: state that can occur after a prolonged period of time without cognitive engagement or practice with using one's typical thinking skills.

Cognitive symptoms: changes in thinking skills, including attention and concentration, learning, memory, executive functioning, language, and processing speed.

Compensatory strategies: techniques that can be employed to adjust to and work around existing difficulties.

Computed tomography (CT) scan: scan generated by the computer processing of many x-ray measurements taken from different angles. CT scans allow medical providers to see cross-sections of the brain or other parts of the body.

Concussion: temporary change in brain functioning or the ability for the brain to do its job when forces from an impact or other type of injury reach the brain. Medically, concussion is defined as the mildest form of brain injury, also referred to as a mild traumatic brain injury, that meets all the following criteria: loss of consciousness (if present) lasting for less than 30 minutes, posttraumatic amnesia (if present) lasting for less than 24 hours, Glasgow Coma Scale score ranging from 13 to 15 and no structural abnormalities seen on standard neuroimaging such as a brain CT scan.

Contact sports: sports in which physical contact is more likely, such as American football, hockey, soccer, or basketball.

Continuous positive airway pressure (CPAP): device used to manage obstructive sleep apnea and other conditions by keeping the airway open to avoid interruptions in breathing.

Contusions: focal bruising that occurs when blood vessels are ruptured or damaged.

Convergence insufficiency: condition in which the eyes have difficulty coordinating the movements necessary to focus on objects.

Counseling: form of treatment carried out by a mental health counselor or other mental health provider that is usually short-term.

Cranial nerves: bundles of brain cells that work together to carry out specific functions involving the head, face, and other body parts.

CT (computed tomography): scan generated by the computer processing of many x-ray measurements taken from different angles. CT scans allow medical providers to see cross-sections of the brain or other parts of the body.

Dementia: progressive loss in cognitive functioning that makes it difficult for a person to carry out daily tasks and maintain independence.

Depersonalization: sensation of being outside one's own body or feeling detached from oneself.

Depression: low mood or loss of interest in activities, among other symptoms, associated with distress and/or functional impairment.

Detachment: emotional numbing or disconnection in the context of relationships with others.

Diffuse axonal injury: stretching and shearing of axons within the brain, common after high-speed motor vehicle accidents.

Dissociative experiences: disruption to or lack of continuity in the normal experience of consciousness, memory, identity, emotions, or perceptions.

Dix-Hallpike maneuver: maneuver used by doctors to assess benign paroxysmal positional vertigo. The patient is asked to rapidly switch from a sitting to a lying position while turning their head from side to side.

Dry needling: treatment in which small needles are placed into trigger points within muscle tissue to release tightness and relieve pain.

Dyslexia: specific learning disorder affecting reading.

Dysphoria: unpleasant emotional state that involves low mood.

Emergency medical technicians (EMTs): medically trained first responders responsible for stabilizing and transporting patients to the hospital during medical emergencies such as motor vehicle accidents, strokes, and heart attacks.

Endocrine system: network of glands and organs that regulate a variety of bodily functions.

Endocrinologist: doctor who specializes in problems of the endocrine system.

Endorphins: chemicals the body releases that make you feel energized.

Epley maneuver: maneuver that involves having a patient lie and hold their head in various positions to help the inner ear crystals (called otoliths) return to their correct location within the ear.

Executive functions: set of cognitive skills including one's ability to engage in goal-directed behavior, planning, set shifting, organization, and self-monitoring of behaviors and emotions.

Exposure therapy: psychological treatment that reduces responses to feared situations through a series of graded exposures.

Eye movement desensitization and reprocessing (EDMR): form of psychotherapy that is effective in treating posttraumatic stress disorder and related conditions.

Family and Medical Leave Act (FMLA): law that provides protections for workers who need to take time off work for a variety of reasons, including after an injury.

Frustration tolerance: one's ability to manage frustration and cope during acutely stressful situations.

Genetics: pertaining to the genetic or inherited properties of a living thing.

GFAP: protein marker that may be used to identify who will need a CT scan after a suspected traumatic brain injury.

Glasgow Coma Scale (GCS): tool used to estimate the severity of a brain injury, widely used in emergency settings and in traumatic brain injury research.

Glaucoma: group of eye diseases characterized by loss of vision resulting from increased pressure within the eye.

Glucose: simple sugar that is a key energy source in humans and other organisms.

Growth hormone: hormone involved in the physical development of children; injury can result in a reduction that is perceived as a decrease in energy or concentration.

Half-life: time it takes for the concentration of a medication to decrease by half within the body.

Head injury: physical injury to the head or scalp.

HIPAA: Health Insurance Portability and Accountability Act, a law that protects patients' right to privacy.

Home sleep test: sleep study conducted in the comfort of one's own home that assesses breathing during sleep but is not as accurate or comprehensive as a polysomnography study.

Hypersomnia: condition that results in excessive sleepiness or spending more time sleeping than is typical.

Hypoglycemia: low blood sugar level.

Individualized Education Program (IEP): plan that outlines formal academic adjustments/accommodations to provide individualized support for students with learning problems, concentration difficulties, intellectual disability, and a host of other conditions who may require extra support in an academic environment.

Inflammatory cascade: series of chemical signals that are carried out within the body in response to stress, injury, or infection.

Inflammatory proteins: proteins that are elevated within the body when the body is responding to stress, injury, or infection.

Insomnia: psychological condition characterized by difficulty falling or staying asleep or difficulties with awakening throughout the night or earlier than desired, resulting in significant impairment in daily functioning and/or significant distress.

Interdisciplinary concussion clinic: outpatient clinic setting in which medical professionals from different disciplines work together to evaluate and treat patients with concussion.

Interdisciplinary team: group of medical professionals from different disciplines who work together to evaluate and treat patients.

Learning disabilities: difficulties with academic skills in reading, writing, or mathematics that do not improve with standard academic supports; also called learning disorders or specific learning disorders.

Learning disorder: difficulty with academic skills in reading, writing, or mathematics that do not improve with standard academic support; also called learning disability or specific learning disorder.

Lidocaine: numbing medication that can be applied to the skin or injected.

Magnetic resonance imaging (MRI): computerized scan that uses a large magnet and radio waves to produce detailed cross-sectional images of internal organs such as the brain.

Massage: physical manipulation (rubbing and kneading) of muscles or joints to reduce tension or pain.

Medication-overuse headaches: headaches that are caused from using over-the-counter headache medications for a prolonged period of time; also called rebound headaches.

Melatonin: hormone produced by the body that helps signal to the body that it is time to sleep; can also be taken as a supplement.

Microtubules: structural supports of brain cells (neurons).

Migraine: headache associated with other signs or symptoms, including nausea or sensitivity to sound or light.

Mild cognitive impairment (MCI): changes in cognitive functioning without significant associated impairment in activities of daily living.

Mild traumatic brain injury: the mildest form of brain injury, the technical definition requires all these criteria and the absence of abnormalities seen on standard structural imaging such as a brain CT scan. Some researchers use only part of the criteria above when using the term mild traumatic brain injury in their studies (such as only using the Glasgow Coma Scale). It is important to clarify exactly what criteria are being used when this term is applied.

Mindfulness: mental state or practice that involves continually bringing one's awareness back to the present moment in a nonjudgmental way.

Mindfulness-based strategies: strategies that help teach or implement aspects of mindfulness.

Mindfulness-based stress reduction: program that has been shown to help individuals manage chronic pain through learning strategies to root down into the present moment and accept difficult circumstances without judgment.

Moderate traumatic brain injury: a brain injury that meets any of the following criteria: loss of consciousness lasting between 30 minutes and 24 hours, posttraumatic amnesia lasting from 1 to 7 days, Glasgow Coma Scale score ranging from 9 to 12.

Mood: emotional state such as feeling happy, angry, or sad.

Motor functioning: extent of ability within the body's movement systems.

Muscle tension headache: headache caused by tightness within muscles of the neck, shoulder, head, or face.

Musculoskeletal: involving the muscles or skeleton.

Nerve cells: cells that typically contain a cell body, axon, and dendrites and communicate with other cells through synapses; also called neurons.

Neural plasticity: the brain's ability to make the new connections necessary for learning and to adapt to changes following injury.

Neuroimaging: general term used to describe different methods for taking pictures of the brain, such as computed tomography (CT) and magnetic resonance imaging (MRI).

Neurologic examination: evaluation carried out by a neurologist that involves assessing orientation, cranial nerves, reflexes, coordination, sensation, and strength.

Neurologist: physician with expertise in brain-based and nervous system medical disorders who has a medical degree and specialty residency training in neurologic disorders.

Neurons: cells that typically contain a cell body, axon, and dendrites and communicate with other cells through synapses; also called nerve cells.

Neuropathic pain: pain that arises from dysfunction within the somatosensory pathways; can be a complication of diabetes.

Neuropsychiatrist: psychiatrist (medical doctor with doctoral and residency training) who has undergone specialized fellowship training in conditions affecting the central nervous system and brain–behavior relationships.

Neuropsychologist: clinical psychologist with a doctoral degree and specialized fellowship training who focuses on the evaluation and treatment of brain-based cognitive and behavioral issues.

Nonsteroidal anti-inflammatory drugs (NSAIDs): group of medications that reduce pain and/or inflammation and are available over the counter or by prescription in higher doses or strengths.

Nystagmus: abnormal eye movements that can occur when the head is thrust in different directions during evaluation or when damage to the vestibular system has occurred.

Obstructive sleep apnea: sleep disorder characterized by recurrent periods in which breathing is disrupted either partially or fully, resulting in reduced oxygen saturation and/or sleep disturbances.

Occipital nerve block: procedure in which lidocaine is injected into the back of the head beneath the surface of the scalp to help relieve muscle tension and headaches.

Occupational therapist: medical professional with graduate training involving practical clinical experience who focuses on assessment and rehabilitation of functional activities and has an understanding of how physical, cognitive, or emotional disturbances associated with an injury may impact daily functioning.

Oriented: state of awareness that is often assessed by asking a person if they know their name, their location, the date/time, and possibly other information, such as who the current president is.

Orthostatic intolerance: when an individual experiences symptoms upon standing or being upright that are relieved when reclining or lying down.

Otoliths: small crystals within the inner ear structures used by the body to detect linear movement and acceleration.

Palming: exercise that involves lightly placing the palms of the hands over the eyes for short periods of time to allow the eyes and eye muscles to fully relax.

Parasympathetic nervous system: part of the body's nervous system that is responsible for conserving energy by slowing heart rate, relaxing muscles in the gastrointestinal tract, and increasing intestinal glandular activity; often referred to as the "rest-and-digest" system.

Parkinson's disease: neurodegenerative movement disorder characterized by tremor, rigidity, and motor slowing in addition to other physical, emotional, and cognitive symptoms.

Pediatrician: physician who focuses on the growth and development of children and adolescents as well as evaluation and management of common illnesses and injuries in children and adolescents.

Pencil pushups: visual therapy technique used to treat convergence insufficiency in which a pencil (or similar object) is used; the patient practices focusing on the object and maintaining focus on the object as it is brought from midline distance in toward the nose.

Peripheral: within a medical context, referring to the peripheral nervous system (outside of the brain and spinal cord). When discussing dizziness or vertigo, refers to structures in the inner ear.

Persisting symptoms after concussion: when symptoms of concussion persist beyond the initial weeks to months following injury; also called post-concussive syndrome, post-concussion syndrome, or post-concussional syndrome.

Pharmacist: medical professional with extensive training (typically a doctoral degree) focused on how to safely prepare and administer medications and how to discuss side effects and drug–drug interactions with the individuals taking those medications.

Pharmacological: referring to medication.

Physiatrist: a medical doctor specializing in Physical medicine & rehabilitation.

Physical medicine & rehabilitation (PM&R): a specialty of medicine that focuses on recovery from orthopedic or neurologic injuries.

Physical therapist: medical professional with a doctoral degree and practical training focused on the evaluation and treatment or rehabilitation of physical injuries using a variety of techniques to help reduce pain levels and increase range of motion.

Physical therapy: care that focuses on improving quality of life by optimizing physical ability and movement and reducing pain levels.

Physician assistant: medical professional with master's-level training who can assist with diagnosis and patient care under the supervision of a physician.

Polysomnography (PSG): diagnostic study usually performed overnight at an outpatient sleep clinic in which the breathing patterns and electrical activity within an individual's brain are recorded during sleep.

Polytrauma: injury or damage to multiple body parts and organ systems.

Post-concussional syndrome: lack of recovery from concussion within the typical time frame; better described as persisting symptoms after concussion.

Post-concussion syndrome: persistence of concussion symptoms beyond the initial weeks to months following injury; better described as persistent symptoms after concussion.

Post-concussive headaches: headaches that begin within 7 days of a concussion; also called acute posttraumatic headaches.

Post-concussive syndrome: persistence of concussion symptoms beyond the initial weeks to months following injury; better described as persistent symptoms after concussion.

Posttraumatic amnesia: period of time after a traumatic brain injury during which a person is not able to form new memories.

Posttraumatic stress disorder (PTSD): psychiatric condition that can arise when an individual is exposed to a horrific or life-threatening situation or observes another in such a situation.

Postural hypotension: form of low blood pressure that occurs upon sitting up or standing; also called orthostatic hypotension.

Postural tachycardia syndrome (POTS): disorder of autonomic dysregulation that results in symptoms that occur when the patient is upright or standing that are relieved when lying down.

Prevalence: number of people within a population who have a condition within a specific duration of time (i.e., how common a condition is).

Primary injury: in the context of blast injury, an injury that occurs when a blast wave from an explosion directly transmits force to the brain, disrupting brain tissue.

Processing speed: cognitive domain that refers to the speed of one's thinking (i.e., how fast a person can understand or process information).

Progressive muscle relaxation: a guided relaxation technique which involves alternating muscle tension and relaxation.

Prophylactic medication: medication used to prevent the onset of a particular illness state.

Proteins: large molecules that perform a variety of functions within the human body.

Psychiatrist: medical doctor with specialized residency training in the diagnosis and treatment of mental conditions.

Psychotherapy: treatment for mental health conditions that is conducted by a licensed clinical psychologist or other mental health provider.

Quaternary injury: a blast-related injury that is not due to primary, secondary, or tertiary blast mechanisms and may include injuries such as burns, smoke inhalation, or exposure to toxic chemicals.

Rebound headaches: headaches that are caused from using over-the-counter headache medications for a prolonged period of time; also called medication-overuse headaches.

Red flags: symptoms that raise concern for more significant illness or injury.

Rescue medication: medication that is prescribed to be taken as needed at the onset of a particular medical event.

Restless legs syndrome: sleep disorder characterized by an urge to move legs at night and is often accompanied by periodic leg movements during sleep.

Return to duty: standardized process by which military personnel may return to their service duties following a concussive injury.

Rotational injury: specific type of brain injury that results when forces hitting the head or body cause the head and neck to spin around.

Saccule: inner ear structure that contains sensory cells that translate head movements (linear accelerations and head tilts in the vertical plane) into neural signals that are interpreted by the brain.

School psychologist: clinical psychologist with a doctoral degree who specializes in behavior and cognition in the context of school.

Secondary injury: in the context of blast injury, an injury that occurs when a blast displaces shrapnel or other objects at high speeds, which then hit the head.

Second impact syndrome: condition in which an individual sustains a second brain injury shortly after sustaining an initial brain injury, which can result in serious injury or death thought to be due to diffuse swelling of the brain.

Selective serotonin reuptake inhibitors (SSRIs): medications that increase levels of serotonin within the brain; SSRIs are the most commonly prescribed class of antidepressant medications.

Self-monitoring: ability to notice and manage aspects of one's own behavior.

Semicircular canals: tubes within the inner ear that contain fluid; their displacement helps transmit information to the brain about when the head is turning or moving in an angular motion.

Serotonin: neurotransmitter (or chemical messenger) that plays a role in stabilizing mood, sleep, and digestive processes.

Serotonin-norepinephrine reuptake inhibitors (SNRIs): class of antidepressant medications that increase levels of serotonin and norepinephrine within the brain; used to treat disorders such as depression, anxiety, and neuropathic pain.

Severe traumatic brain injury: the most severe form of brain injury. It meets any of the following criteria: loss of consciousness lasting for longer than 24 hours, posttraumatic amnesia lasting longer than 7 days, Glasgow Coma Scale score ranging from 3 to 8.

Slow-wave sleep: the deepest phase of non–rapid eye movement sleep.

Specific learning disorder: condition that is diagnosed based on persisting difficulties with academic skills in reading, writing, or mathematics that do not improve with standard academic supports.

Speech/language pathology: the field of a speech/language pathologist, a medical professional trained in diagnosis and treatment of communication, language, and speech/swallowing disorders.

Sport Concussion Assessment Tool—5th Edition (SCAT5): assessment tool that clinicians use to evaluate for concussion.

Sports medicine physician: physician with specialty training in musculoskeletal injuries and common medical conditions that affect those with a physically active lifestyle and participation in athletics.

Sports neurologist: neurologist with specialty training in brain-based and nervous system medical disorders and specialized fellowship training in sport-related neurologic injuries.

Sports neuropsychologist: clinical neuropsychologist with specialized training/experience in applying knowledge of brain–behavior relationships to the evaluation and treatment of sports-related brain injury.

Steroids: chemicals present in the body that reduce inflammation or reduce activity within the body's immune system; can also be taken in the form of medication.

Stimulant medication: medication that increases one's level of alertness or arousal and can help individuals with attention and/or concentration problems.

Stroke: reduced blood supply to the brain tissue resulting from blockage within blood vessels or bleeding within the brain.

Subconcussive injury: head injury that does not reach the severity threshold of a concussion or mild traumatic brain injury.

Substance P: inflammatory protein secreted by nerves and inflammatory cells.

Sumatriptan: medication that is often prescribed as a rescue medication for migraine; part of the triptan class of medications.

Tau: protein found predominantly in brain cells that plays an important role in stabilizing microtubules, which are part of the cell's structural system.

Tauopathies: conditions in which the primary characteristic of disease is thought to be problematic buildup of a protein in the brain known as tau.

Temperature caloric testing: procedure in which eye movements are measured in response to either cold water or warm air being injected into the ear; also called cold water caloric testing.

Tension-type headaches: headaches caused by tightness within muscles of the neck, shoulder, head, or face.

Tertiary injury: in the context of blast injury, an injury that occurs when an explosion results in a person being thrown to the ground or into another stationary object at high speed.

Testosterone: hormone that plays a role in energy, drive, and motivation.

Tilt-table test: test used to understand why a patient is experiencing fainting or lightheadedness.

Tract: bundle of axons that fire together to send messages throughout the brain.

Traumatic brain injury: form of acquired brain injury due to an external force.

Traumatic encephalopathy syndrome (TES): collection of symptoms and diagnostic findings someone with chronic traumatic encephalopathy may have before death.

Trigger point injections: treatment in which lidocaine (a numbing medication) is injected into tender muscle areas to help relieve muscle tightness and reduce pain.

Triptans: class of medications used in the rescue treatment of migraines.

Tympanic membrane: cone-shaped structure that distinguishes the external ear from the middle ear and transmits sound vibrations to assist with hearing; commonly referred to as the eardrum.

UCHL-1: protein marker that may be used to identify who will need a CT scan after a suspected traumatic brain injury.

Utricle: inner ear structure that contains sensory cells that translate head movements (linear accelerations and head tilts in the horizontal plane) into neural signals that are interpreted by the brain.

Vascular dementia: condition that can result in a wide variety of cognitive problems, including reduced executive functioning and processing speed, when blood flow to the brain is reduced either suddenly (as in major strokes) or more gradually over time (as is in small vessel ischemic disease).

Vertigo: sensation of dizziness that feels as though the room were spinning.

Vestibular system: system of body parts that work together to help the body maintain its balance and sense of direction.

Video nystagmogram (VNG): technology that uses infrared goggles to allow vestibular specialists to identify the cause of vestibular dysfunction by assessing the inner ear in conjunction with eye movements.

Virtual reality goggles: goggles that project lifelike images or situations.

Virtual reality therapy: type of exposure therapy used in treating PTSD in which the patient wears goggles that project lifelike images or situations that induce fear.

Vocational rehabilitation specialist: professional who has training in identifying the specific requirements of different jobs and helping individuals find appropriate jobs based on their interests and abilities or providing support for those reentering the job force following a period of disability or leave.

Whiplash injury: colloquial term used to describe neck injury caused by rapid acceleration and deceleration.

Workers' compensation: system that works to protect injured employees from some of the negative financial consequences of an injury sustained while at work by providing up to two-thirds of any lost wages during a period of medical leave and covering the costs of associated medical care.

X-ray: a type of electromagnetic radiation that is used to produce images of the body's internal structures.

ABOUT *BRAIN & LIFE*® AND THE AMERICAN ACADEMY OF NEUROLOGY

Brain & Life® is the only magazine and website focused on the intersection of brain health and neurologic disease. A print subscription to *Brain & Life* (six issues a year) is available for free to anyone residing in the United States. Visit *BrainandLife.org* to subscribe or read stories on brain science, brain health and wellness, and living well with neurologic disorders.

Brain & Life is an official publication of the American Academy of Neurology (AAN). Founded in 1948, the AAN represents more than 38,000 members who are neurologists and neuroscience professionals and is dedicated to promoting the highest-quality patient-centered neurologic care. A neurologist is a doctor with specialized training in diagnosing, treating, and managing disorders of the brain and nervous system such as Alzheimer's disease, stroke, migraine, multiple sclerosis, concussion, Parkinson's disease, and epilepsy. For more information about the American Academy of Neurology, visit *AAN.com*.

INDEX

For the benefit of digital users, indexed terms that span two pages (e.g., 52–53) may, on occasion, appear on only one of those pages.

Tables, figures, and boxes are indicated by *t*, *f*, and *b* following the page number